PREVENT

Suggested Activities to Motivate the Teaching of Elementary Safety

AUTHOR

ZANE A. SPENCER

FLINT, MICHIGAN

PUBLISHED BY
EDUCATIONAL SERVICE, INC.
P. O. Box 219
Stevensville, Michigan 49127

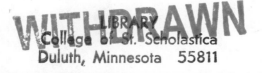

Copyright 1975©
EDUCATIONAL SERVICE, INC.
P.O. Box 219
Stevensville, Michigan 49127
Printed in U.S.A.
ISBN #89273-115-X

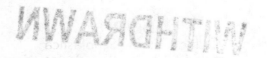

TABLE OF CONTENTS

SECTION III: TRAVELING SAFELY BY FOOT, CAR, BUS AND AIR

SECTION IV: LIVING SAFELY IN THE CITY

SECTION V: LIVING SAFELY ON THE FARM

SECTION VI: SAFETY IN PLAY AND ON VACATIONS

SECTION VII: FIRST AID

vi

SECTION X: REVIEW AND REINFORCEMENT ACTIVITIES

INTRODUCTION

PREVENT is another in a series of handbooks published by Educational Service, Inc. to provide teachers with practical ideas and activities that enrich their teaching programs.

PREVENT is written for the elementary school teacher to provide new and interesting habits among their students. Ours is a complex world and there are many ways in which accidents can happen. Through PREVENT, ideas, games and independent activities are offered to help students become alert to the ways in which accidents can be prevented and avoided. As a result of this exposure, it is hoped that they will be better prepared to meet most of the emergencies that they might encounter.

Each classroom tested activity includes a description of all necessary materials and preparations, and an example of how the activity may be presented to the class. The materials was condensed as much as possible, in order to include many different activities within the space limitations of a truly functional handbook.

PREVENT is a handbook written especially for teachers who recognize that learning to live safely is a worthy goal for everyone now and in the future.

SECTION I: Safety in the Home

A great many minor and major accidents occur in homes. Children should be aware of the reasons such accidents happen and to learn that they can help prevent them. This section is designed to help them explore and think about their homes. This is where they live and where safety really begins for them.

1. HOME ACCIDENT SURVEY

*
**1. HOME ACCIDENT SURVEY
(Grades K-8)

    A. Preparation and Materials: Write on the board or prepare a chart listing the most common types of home accidents.

    Example:

Home Accident Survey	
Falls	||||| |||
Burns	||
Cuts		
Bumps	||||| |||||	
Bruises	||||| ||||| ||
Sprains	||
Broken Bones		
Fires	
Poison	

*This activity is available in Prevent Volume I of the **Spice**™ Duplicating Masters.
This activity is available in Prevent Volume II of the **Spice™ Duplicating Masters.

B. Introduction to the Class: Today, we are going to make a home accident survey. How many of you have had some kind of accident in your home? Has someone else in your family had an accident in your home? Let's talk about home accidents and try to find out which kinds of accidents seem to occur most frequently in our class. I have made a chart (or list on the board) of the most common types of accidents. Mark, would you like to keep score?

C. Variation: Older children could be asked to compile a series of accident anecdotes. When they have finished, each student could read his or her anecdote and the scorekeeper could chart the results.

*
**2. ANALYZING ACCIDENTS (Grades K-8)

A. Preparation and Materials: Write a list of questions adapted to grade level on the chalk board.

Example:

1. What happened and why?
2. What happened before the accident?
3. What were the psychological or human factors?
4. What was wrong in the environment?
5. What could be done to prevent a repeat of that particular accident?

B. Introduction to the Class: Near accidents are far more common than actual accidents. Today, we are going to try to analyze some close calls as well as actual accidents. Let's see if we can find some clues for accident prevention in our homes.

—4—

To get us started I would like to tell you about a near accident at our house last night. I put some books on the stairs. I was planning to take them up later, but I forgot they were there. I stumbled over them and almost fell up the stairs on my face. How could that almost accident have been prevented?

Yes, Jimmy, I should have put the books away in the first place. Stairs should never be cluttered with anything someone might fall on.

Can you think of a way that a worse accident could have happened?

Right, Lindy, someone could have been coming down the stairs.

*3. IT DOESN'T BELONG (Grades K-3)

A. Preparation and Materials: Prepare a duplicated sheet with several safety ideas pictured. Include some unsafe home practices.

Example:

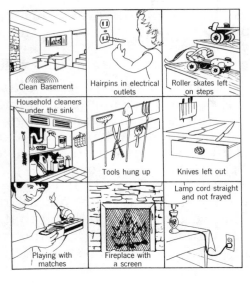

—5—

*This activity is available in Prevent Volume I of the **Spice**™ Duplicating Masters.

B. Introduction to the Class: Now that we have been talking about safety in our homes, let's see if we can spot some unsafe ideas on the paper I have given you. What about the first picture, John? Is that basement safe from fire hazards? Yes, a clean basement is safe. We will leave that picture alone.

What about the second picture? Should anyone put a hairpin in an electrical outlet? No, that picture does not belong in a safe house. Let's put an X on it.

C. Variation: Safe and unsafe situations could be collected from magazines and mounted on tagboard. Use the reading pocket chart as a game board and let the children choose those situations which do not belong. Each child could be allowed to explain why he feels the picture he removes does not belong in the game.

*4. TIC TAC SAFETY (Grades 1-4)

A. Preparation and Materials: Prepare a duplicated sheet similar to the example. Also have on hand a supply of blank duplicated Tic Tac Safety grids. The students will need pencils.

B. Introduction to the Class: Many boys and girls have accidents at home because they forget that there are some things in every home that they should not touch or that some things need to be handled with special care. I have a Tic Tac Safety game for you to play today. Read each word carefully. If it is a toy you know is safe for you to play with, put a circle on it.

If a word does not tell you that it is a toy, put an X on it. That will remind you that those things are for dads and mothers. If you handle

*This activity is available in Prevent Volume I of the **Spice**™ Duplicating Masters.

them at all, handle them with special care.

Can anyone guess which rows will be winners? Will the X rows win or will it be the O rows?

Yes, you'll be a winner and help avoid home accidents, too, if you know that circles make the Tic Tac Safety row.

Now, find the winning row on this game.

When you have finished, come up and take a blank Tic Tac Safety grid. See if you can make your own game. If you need help with spelling, use your dictionary or come up and ask me.

Tomorrow, we will exchange papers and play the games you have made. Remember, your Tic Tac Safety row does not have to be like the one I made. It can be any horizontal, vertical, or diagonal row. See what you can do.

Example:

dolls	guns	pills
ammunition	balls	knives
razor blades	matches	bike

**5. ONE STEP BEYOND (Grades 4-8)

A. Preparation and Materials: Students will need pencils and a duplicated sheet containing three columns. Column A should include a list of several home appliances and other consumer products which have caused accidents in homes.

Resource material, such as government publications and appliance operating manuals, would be helpful but not necessary especially if students are allowed to take the assignment home and discuss it with their parents.

Examples for Column A:

1. Microwave oven
2. Ladder
3. Glass doors
4. T.V. set
5. Power lawn mower
6. Sunlamp
7. Fireplace
8. Kitchen appliances operating simultaneously
9. Cleaning supplies
10. Pesticides

B. Introduction to the Class: Because we spend a great deal of time at home, it is easy to take things for granted. These things are there. We use them and that's it. Seldom do we take the time to really think about safety. This is the main reason there are so many home accidents.

Today, we are going to take a critical look at some of the things we see and use everyday in our homes. I have listed several items in Column A. Think about each one. What type of accident might result? What type of injury could be in-

This activity is available in Prevent Volume II of the **Spice™ Duplicating Masters.

volved? Would you fall, get burned, cut or maybe poisoned? Put your answer in Column B. This column will probably be very easy for you to fill in once you stop and think about it.

But now, let your thinking go One Step Beyond. What safety precaution might be taken to avoid an accident with the item listed in Column A? This answer goes in Column C and it might be as simple as: "Read the instructions in the operating manual carefully." Other answers might involve using your common sense, for example: "Never have a loose throw rug in front of a glass door."

You may use the resource material, or you may take the assignment home and ask your parents to help you fill in the blanks. They will probably be glad to play the One Step Beyond game with you.

*6. DRAMATIZING DANGER (Grades K-8)

A. Preparation and Materials: Prepare a set of accident situation cards.

Example:

Accident Situation: Poison

You discover your baby brother crawling toward a puddle of something spilled on the bathroom floor. You don't know what has been spilled. What would you do?

You may also want to color code a set of possible solutions for children who need extra help in knowing what to do.

*This activity is available in Prevent Volume I of the Spice™ Duplicating Masters.

Example:

Possible Solution: Poison

Stop baby from tasting the spill because it might be poison. Call your mother.

Older children may be allowed to write their own set of cards or they may wish to write plays or skits.

B. Directions to the Class: I will choose two (or number called for in situation) people and give them an accident situation. They will read the card and we will give them a minute or two to decide how they want to act out the situation. They will enact the dangerous situation and show what they think is the right thing to do. Remember there may be more than one right solution. After each little drama we will talk about other possibilities.

**7. A MINUTE OR LESS (Grades 4-8)

A. Preparation and Materials: Prepare or allow a group of students to prepare a set of word cards using two or three key words from each of the rules or safety precautions learned about electricity.

Example:

FIRE ELECTRICAL WATER

**This activity is available in Prevent Volume II of the Spice™ Duplicating Masters.

B. Directions to the Class: Now that you have finished the key word cards on electricity, we will use them to play a review game called A Minute or Less. This is the way it goes. If Matt drew the card "FIRE ELECTRICAL WATER", he would be given A Minute or Less to come up with the rule that would use all three of these key words.

Can you do it, Matt?

Yes, "Never throw water on an electrical fire" would be a right answer.

Other Examples:

Word Card: DANGER KITE ELECTRIC

Answer: There is danger if you fly a kite near electric wires.

Word Card: METAL CORD

Answer: It is dangerous to hang electric cords on metal objects.

Word Card: STORM TREE HIDE

Answer: Never hide under a tree during a storm.

C. Variations:

1. Use this technique as a writing exercise. Write the word combinations on the board and let each child try each set of words. Share the results after each exercise.

2. This technique could be used as a review after any area of safety has been covered.

**8. SAFETY EYE ON CORDS (Grades 4-8)

A. Preparation and Materials: Prepare a duplicated sheet similar to the example. An old electric cord and a knife will also be needed.

This activity is available in Prevent Volume II of the **Spice™ Duplicating Masters.

Example:

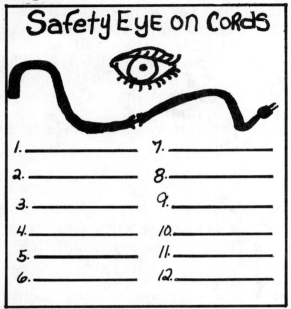

B. Introduction to the Class: I'm sure many of you have heard that faulty electrical wires can cause fires. Have you ever wondered why? Let's cut this old cord apart and see if we can find the answer. (Cut the cord and discuss how electricity must make a complete circuit. Point out that electricity always follows the easiest path and if there is a short circuit the electricity goes there instead of where it is supposed to go. Discuss how this could cause a fire.)

Can you think how electric cords might have a short circuit now that we have taken this one apart and discussed it. Yes, Randy, if the insulation is frayed it could cause a short circuit. This is why it is a good idea to check electric cords in your house every so often.

On your Safety Eye paper, make a list of all the things in your house that use electricity. Tonight, when you go home from school, check the cords you have listed. See if any of them are frayed. If you find one, tell your mom or dad. They can fix it or buy a new one. Your Safety Eye might prevent a fire at your house.

9. SAFETY SOAPS (Grades 3-8)

A. Preparation and Materials: Each child will need a bar of soap and a knife.

B. Introduction to the Class: For more years than we can count, men have whittled and carved to pass the time and to express their feelings in works of art. Cave men carved stories on their cave walls using primitive tools. Today, our tools are perfected and probably much sharper. However, any type of carving tool can be dangerous. Today, we are going to learn to carve safely with a knife.

You each have a bar of soap. We will call your carving a Safety Soap. You may choose to carve an animal or a person. You may even choose to design a bar of soap that is shaped differently. What you make is up to you. Our main purpose today is to learn how to use a sharp knife safely.

There are three very important safety rules to follow. I will write them on the board (or put them on a poster). Let's discuss each rule before we begin. Tell why you think each rule is a good one.

1. Make sure you have plenty of room.
2. Never leave a knife blade out when not in use. (Jackknife blades should be closed.)
3. Always stroke away from you.

C. Variations: These activities could be used effectively with younger children. The teacher could demonstrate the safe way to use a knife.

1. Make applesauce. Correlate with a visit to the local apple orchard.
2. Make vegetable soup. Correlate with a study on taste, smell and touch.

10. SHARP DISPLAY (Grades 4-8)

A. Preparation and Materials: Provide a bulletin board or display case. Students will need resource materials and materials for making a chart.

B. Introduction to the Class: Sharp objects cause a great many home accidents. Can you think of some sharp objects that might cause an accident in your home? Right, Mickey, knives are one of the major culprits.

Yes, Janice, razor blades and scissors would be two more sharp objects that might cause accidents. (Continue the discussion letting the students describe any sharp objects they think would cause an accident.)

Do you suppose you could chart some statistics on the hazards of sharp objects? It would be interesting to know just how many knife accidents did happen last year, for example. Go to the library and ask the librarian to help you seek some statistics. Put your findings on this chart and use this board for a Sharp Display. You may cut pictures from magazines or draw them. You might also use real, sharp objects if you can mount them easily and safely.

As you work on your Sharp Display, keep in mind all of the things that might be done to avoid accidents involving sharp objects in the home. Making sure that throw rugs are anchored well would be one way to prevent falling on a sharp object, wouldn't it?

11. SAFETY GIFT FOR DAD (Grades K-3)

A. Preparation and Materials: Each child will need an orange juice can, matchbook covers or pictures from magazines, glue, scissors, rickrack or braid, varnish or shellac.

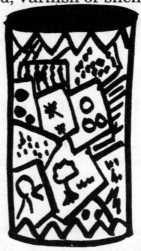

B. Introduction to the Class: Razor blades are very sharp, aren't they? Your fathers need them in the house so they can shave their whiskers, but dads are grown up and they know the safe way to handle them.

What do you think would happen if your dad accidentally left a razor blade on the sink or someplace where a little brother or sister might find it? Yes, Bonnie, I agree. I think a little one would pick it up to see what it is and they would probably get cut.

Let's use these supplies to make a safety gift for dad. Let's make him a container for his old razor blades. I'm sure dad will be very pleased that you are thinking about safety in your home.

C. Directions:

1. Glue the matchbook covers or pictures to the can.

2. Glue rickrack or braid around the top and/ or bottom for decoration.

3. When the glue is dry, spray with varnish or paint with shellac.

D. Correlation: This activity could be correlated with a gift for Father's Day.

*12. FOLLOW THE DOTS TO FIRE SAFETY (Grades 1-4)

A. Preparation and Materials: Prepare a duplicated sheet similar to the example. The students will need pencils. Crayons are optional.

Example:

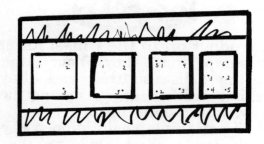

Connect the dots in each block. Then turn your paper upside down to find out what to do if your clothes catch on fire.

*This activity is available in Prevent Volume I of the **Spice**™ Duplicating Masters.

B. Directions to the Class: Sometimes we forget that clothes can catch on fire just as paper can. Some clothes will burn as fast as paper, too.

There are many ways your clothes could catch on fire. Can you think of some of the ways?

Examples:

1. Standing too close to a fireplace or campfire.
2. Playing with matches.
3. Burning trash.
4. Filling gasoline engines, such as lawn mowers, power saws, snowmobiles, etc.

Burns can cause pain, bad scars and even death. To grow up safely, you must know what to do. Today's safety puzzle will give you the magic word. Follow the dots in each block and then turn your paper upside down to see what to do if your clothes catch on fire.

You may color the flames if you like and then when everyone is done, we will talk about the magic word. Perhaps some of you will remember stories you can share. Can you think of an incident where a life was saved because someone knew what to do?

13. SAFE HANDS (Grades K-3)

A. Preparation and Materials: Each child will need a sheet of 12x18 inch colored construction paper. Contrasting construction paper (large enough for children to trace hands onto), scissors, paste and construction paper scraps for match will also be needed.

B. Introduction to the Class: Many home fires are started by children who play with matches. This is very dangerous and today, we are

are going to remind our hands that no matter what, they will not play with matches.

C. Directions:

1. Trace your hands onto your construction paper.

2. Cut out your hands.

3. Paste them on this big sheet of paper.

4. Use the scrap box and cut a pretend match and paste it between your hands like this:

Example:

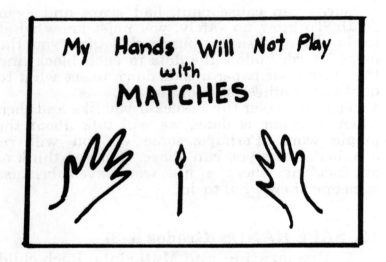

5. You may use your black crayon and print this title on your safety poster.

MY HANDS WILL NOT PLAY WITH MATCHES

(Note: Kindergarten teacher will probably need to do the printing for the children.)

14. JUICY MR. JACK-O'-LANTERN
(Grades K-1)

A. Preparation and Materials: Materials needed are orange construction paper, yellow scraps of construction paper or gold foil wrapping paper, paste, scissors, crayons and a tagboard pumpkin pattern.

Example:

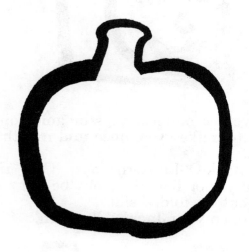

B. Introduction to the Class: Halloween is almost here and Jack-O'-Lanterns are a must for Halloween, aren't they? Today, we are going to make some special Jack-O'-Lanterns. They are safety Jack-O'-Lanterns.

C. Directions:

1. Fold your sheet of orange construction paper in half. (Demonstrate.)

2. Use this pattern and trace the pumpkin on one half of the paper. Be sure to place one side of the pattern on the folded edge.

Example:

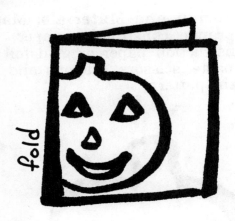

3. Use yellow paper scraps or gold foil wrapping paper to make eyes, nose and mouth. Paste in place.

4. Cut Jack-O'-Lantern out. Cut through your folded paper like this, but be very careful you do not cut the folded side.

5. Now open your Jack-O'-Lantern.

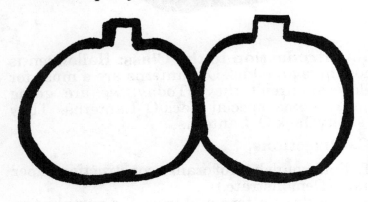

6. On the inside you may draw a candle with your crayons.

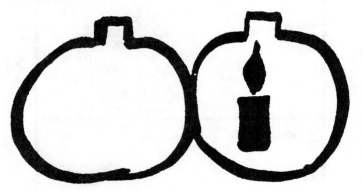

Would you ever put a real candle inside a paper pumpkin or paper Halloween lantern? Why not? Right, Tommy, it could start a fire. Remember that candles should only be put inside juicy cornfield pumpkins so if they fall over, they will go out.

*15. CHRISTMAS TREE, O CHRISTMAS TREE (Grades K-4)

A. Preparation and Materials: Prepare a duplicated sheet similar to the example. The students will need crayons.

B. Introduction to the Class: Look at the picture of the Christmas tree at the top of your paper. It is not a safe tree, is it? Can you name some of the things wrong with it? That's right, Paige. You should never use real candles on a Christmas tree. It is a fire hazard.

Yes, Craig, you found another danger, didn't you? The tree is too close to the fireplace. That is also a fire hazard.

*This activity is available in Prevent Volume I of the **Spice**™ Duplicating Masters.

Example:

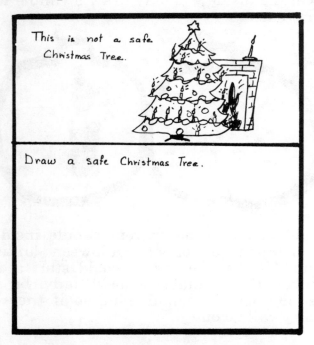

This is not a safe Christmas Tree.

Draw a safe Christmas Tree.

Yes, Lin, a third fire hazard is the fact that the tree has no place for adding water to the trunk.

Now, use the space at the bottom of your paper to draw a safe Christmas tree. Then, when you go home, you might check your own Christmas tree to see if it is a safe tree.

*16. CHECKING UP ON CHRISTMAS (Grades K-8)

A. Preparation and Materials: Older students will need pencils and paper. Younger children may tell their ideas. Poster board will be needed for the chart and felt pens for writing on the chart.

*This activity is available in Prevent Volume I of the **Spice**™ Duplicating Masters.

B. Introduction to the Class: Have you ever noticed how many accidents happen in the home at Christmas time? Remember that there are reasons for accidents. Sometimes, people are careless and sometimes reasons are created when people just don't know simple safety rules. Either way, accidents can spoil a Christmas.

I'd like you to do some Checking Up On Christmas at your house. In what ways do you and your family take precautions to make Christmas safe?

Take some time with your check list. Ask your parents to help you. Then we will organize a classroom Christmas check chart. We will put all of your best ideas on the chart. You may even discover some safety precautions you haven't thought about.

Idea for Decorating Christmas Check-Up Chart: Tack a sparkly Christmas rope around the edge of the chart.

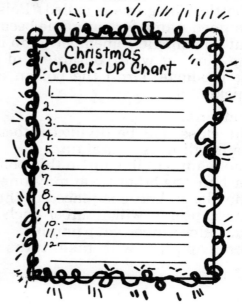

17. POISON GRAB (Grades K-4)

A. Preparation and Materials: A plastic gallon size bleach bottle is needed. Be sure it is rinsed out.

B. Introduction to the Class: Every year many boys and girls are poisoned by drinking household cleaners of some kind. Can you think of some things in your home that might be dangerous?

I have a big bottle here. (Show bleach bottle.) Do you think what was inside this bottle could be poison if someone drank it? Yes, and almost every mother uses bleach to help make the wash whiter. I should think it would taste terrible. Why do you suppose some little boys and girls would try to taste it? Probably they are just curious. Babies try lots of things, don't they? They don't know any better.

Today, we are going to play a game with this bleach bottle. The game is called "Poison Grab." This is a good name for our game because that is just what you should remember to do if you see a little one playing with containers of household cleaning products. Grab the poison away from them quickly.

Directions:

1. The class will be divided into two teams. Each team will have a captain.

2. One team will line up on this boundary line and over here the other team may line up.

3. The bleach bottle is placed in the center.

4. The captains will number each person on their team. Remember your number.

5. The captains will take turns calling a number.

6. The two players (one from each team) who have that number will run to the center and try to grab the bottle. They will try to get back to their team without being tagged. If they do, they get a point for their team. If they don't, the other team gets the point.

7. When all of the numbers have been called, the team with the most points is the winner.

18. READ THE LABEL (Grades 6-8)

A. Preparation and Materials: Several containers and instruction manuals should be on hand for demonstration.

B. Introduction to the Class: Have you ever noticed how many new products and devices are on the market today? Manufacturers are constantly trying to make products, tools and appliances better. This is good for us as consumers, but it does put some extra responsibility on us as far as safety goes. It means that we must always be careful to read the labels and directions before trying new things. For safety's sake we must make this a habit.

To help get you started on the label reading habit, I would like you to read the labels and directions on as many devices and products as you can during the next week. Keep a record of what you read. You will get one point for each name on your list. The person with the most points will be the winner. However, all of you will be winners because you have begun a habit which could save your life someday.

C. Correlation: Correlate this activity with reading, using it to strengthen reading skills. Students could be asked to bring in a different label each day and read it at a specified time.

19. POISON MOBILES (Grades K-8)

A. Preparation and Materials: Have a discussion on the many common household items found under the sink or in medicine chests which might be harmful if swallowed, or in some cases breathed. Ask the children to bring in empty containers of the plastic or cardboard variety.

Examples: Bleach bottles, dish soap, floor wax, ammonia, toilet bowl cleaner, sink cleaner, drain openers, etc. (Wire coat hangers and yarn will also be needed.)

B. Introduction to the Class: Now that we have discussed some common household items that could be poison, let's use some of the plastic containers to make poison mobiles. You may divide into groups to work and when you are finished, we will hang the mobiles from the ceiling. Remember, a mobile must be balanced to hang properly.

Example:

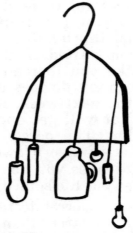

C. Correlation: This activity could be cor related with a math unit on balance.

**20. "O" FOR HELP (Grades K-8)

A. Preparation and Materials: Prepare a duplicated sheet similar to the example. Adapt discussion to grade level. Younger children may be asked to name letters under "O". Put the letters on the chalkboard and then read the safety message for them.

Example:

X	X	O	X	X	O	X	X	O	X	O
R	Z	D	P	T	O	C	F	N	S	O

O	X	X	O	O	X	X	O	X	X	X
T	A	Q	H	A	V	B	N	T	R	E

X	O	X	X	X	O	X	O	X	X	X
D	G	W	Y	P	U	H	P	M	N	C

B. Introduction to the Class: Sometimes, when people want to report a fire or an accident of some kind, they panic. They get so excited they can't remember who to call or what number to dial. This happens to grown-ups, too. It is very hard to remember just what to do when danger is near.

Almost everyone can remember to dial the operator if they need help. This is all right especially if you can tell the operator what kind of help you need and where you need it, but what happens if you dial the operator and can't think of anything to say but "HELP?" Can the operator send help to you?

*This activity is available in Prevent Volume I of the **Spice**™ Duplicating Masters.
This activity is available in Prevent Volume II of the **Spice™ Duplicating Masters.

Yes, she can IF you remember one more very important safety rule. You will find this rule in your safety paper today. Just copy down all of the letters under the O's and you will see the message.

C. Correlation: Correlate with a lesson in letter recognition.

SECTION II: Safety at School

Accidents decrease sharply after children start school. One reason for this is that teachers do teach safety precautions. Safety, like good health practices, must become a habit. This chapter is designed to reinforce safety habits as well as emphasize particular school safety precautions.

1. SAFETY STAR MAN (Grades K-1)

A. Preparation and Materials: This activity works well at the beginning of the school year when classroom safety rules are being discussed. The children will need a sheet of 9x12 inch colored construction paper and chalk.

B. Introduction to the Class: Now that we have talked about our classroom safety rules, we are going to make safety star men. When you are finished I will tack them on the back board. If you remember our safety rules all day, you may take your star man home. If you forget, your star man will have to stay on the board. It must stay there until you can remember our class safety rules for one whole day.

C. Directions: (Demonstrate as you tell the children what to do.)

1. Draw a man with his feet wide apart.
   He's a safety man right from the start.

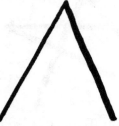

2. Out go his arms, but he doesn't hit.
   He's a safety man. You can bet on it.

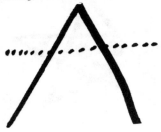

3. He never runs in the room.
   His head won't go boom.
   He bends down low
   To touch his opposite toe.

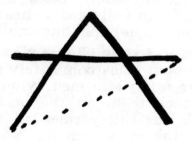

4. Pushing at the drinking fountain is out.
   He knows what safety is all about.
   Now, down once more with the other hand.
   Look, boys and girls, you've made a safety star man.

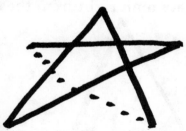

5. Now, can you find a place to give him a happy face?

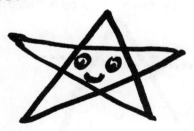

6. Be sure to print your name on the bottom of your paper. (Younger children may need help.)
7. When you have finished, bring your star man to me. I'll put him on the board until it's time to go home.

2. STOP, LOOK, AND CARRY
(Grades K-1)

A. Preparation and Materials: Prepare a tray with several school supplies on it. Include a box of crayons, scissors, jar of paste, pencil, paint brush, a sheet of paper, etc.

The children sit in a circle and the tray is placed in the middle of the circle.

B. Introduction to the Class: Sometimes it doesn't matter how we carry things at school. Sometimes it does matter. Let's see if we can figure out how to carry the school supplies on this tray. I am going to call on someone and ask that person to bring me something. If I call on you, go to the tray, stop, look at what I have asked you to bring me. Pick it up and tell me how you will carry it and why you choose to carry it that way. If it doesn't matter, tell me it doesn't matter.

Billy, you may start. Bring me the sheet of paper. Right, it doesn't matter how we carry a sheet of paper, does it?

Lynn, you may bring me the scissors. Stop, look and tell me how you will carry them. Lightly by the scissor handles with the blades pointing down. Very good. Can you tell me why? Yes, you might fall on the blades and hurt yourself.

After we have gone through the game once, I will put the things back on the tray. This time if I call on someone who decides to carry something in an unsafe way, the rest of you say, STOP, LOOK, AND CARRY. Then I will choose someone to tell why the object should be carried some other way.

*3. SNIPPER SNOOPER (Grades K-1)

A. Preparation and Materials: This activity is designed to give young children cutting practice as well as reinforce the safe way to carry scissors. Materials needed are scissors and crayons. Prepare a duplicated sheet similar to the example.

Example:

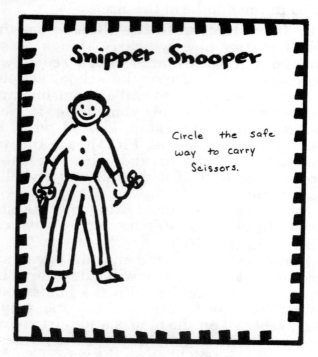

*This activity is available in Prevent Volume I of the **Spice**™ Duplicating Masters.

B. Directions to the Class: This little boy is called Snipper Snooper. Notice he has two pairs of scissors. He is carrying one pair safely. Do you know which pair? Put a circle around the safe way to carry scissors. Put an X on the unsafe way. Jerry, tell us why you put a circle around Snipper Snooper's right hand. Why is the other way unsafe?

Color Snipper Snooper with your crayons and then use your scissors to snip around the edge of your paper. Be very careful to stay in the dark paths like this. (Demonstrate snipping and how to turn the paper as you go around the corner.)

4. SHARP ART (Grades K-8)

A. Preparation and Materials: Students will need a supply of old holiday cards, black crayons, and a sharp scraping tool such as scissor points, a metal nail file, knife or ruler edge.

Discuss the safe use of sharp objects if not done in a previous lesson.

B. Introduction to the Class: We have been talking about the safe way to use sharp objects in the classroom. We know how to hold scissors and we know we should never run with something sharp in our hand. (Adapt review of safety rules to grade level.)

Today, we are going to do a fun art project with sharp objects. I expect each of you to remember and follow the safety rules we discussed. Remember that thinking about safety is easy but not thinking about it can sometimes be very hard on you. It can hurt.

C. Directions: First, select an old holiday card from these on the table. Color the face of your card with a black crayon. (Tables and desks can be protected with newspaper.) Make the black very heavy. Really press down.

Now, take a sharp object and scrape a picture on the card. Note how the colors come through like magic.

*5. "ACCORDION" TO SAFETY
(Grades K-8)

A. Preparation and Materials: Each student will need three sheets of drawing paper, tape, crayons and a felt pen for recording comments. The teacher may take dictation from younger students.

B. Introduction to the Class: We are going to make accordion-folded books today so that you may show some of the things you do at school to help you stay safe. We have talked about several good safety habits to develop. Can you name one, Mary?

Yes, that is a good one. Never run in the room or in the hall because you might fall and hurt yourself. (Adapt discussion to grade level and continue encouraging the students to remember other safety rules.)

Example:
1. Don't push at drinking fountains.
2. Be careful when using glass containers.
3. Don't climb on chairs or tables.
4. Don't push in line.
5. Don't try to carry loads that are too heavy.
6. Don't leave soap on the floor if you drop it.
7. Watch for ice on the playground and sidewalk.

*This activity is available in Prevent Volume I of the **Spice**™ Duplicating Masters.

8. Be careful with sharp objects.

9. Don't put fingers in cracks of doors and desks where they might be pinched.

10. Make sure you have plenty of room if you are playing or working with something that might hurt others. (Bats, or knives, etc.)

C. Directions:

1. Each of you will have three sheets of manila drawing paper. Tape them together end to end like this. (Demonstrate.)

2. Accordion fold the paper into six parts.

3. Label the first section with your title.

"Accordion" To Good Safety Habits
or
My Safety Habits

(NOTE: You might discuss the play on the word accordion and ask children to give examples of other plays on words.)

4. On each of the remaining five pages draw a different picture of something you can do to stay safe at school.

5. Put a comment under each picture. (You may tell me what you want to say and I will write it under the picture for you.)

6. When you finish, we will discuss your work. I may ask one of you to show a picture you have drawn and then ask the class to guess why they think you chose that habit as a safe one. (For example: Don't push at the drinking fountain. Reason it is a good habit: The person drinking might chip his teeth.)

6. BELL RINGER (Grades K-6)

A. Preparation and Materials: A bell is needed. Children may sit or stand in a circle.

B. Introduction to the Class: Today, we are going to play a game called "Bell Ringer." This is a game to help you remember some of the rules that keep you safe at school. What are some of these rules? Walter, do you remember the one about going down the hall safely? (Continue with a brief review of school safety rules.)

C. Directions:

1. I will choose one student to be "It".
2. "It" will stand with his back to the rest of the class.
3. The rest of you will have this bell which you must ring when "It" says "Go".
4. Pass the bell from hand to hand. When "It" calls "Stop", he must then turn around and guess who has the bell.
5. If he guesses right, he exchanges places with that person who then becomes the new "It".
6. If he guesses wrong, the person he calls must show he doesn't have the bell and then give a safety rule correctly. If that person doesn't know a rule, he becomes the new "It". Rules cannot be repeated.
7. The object is not to get caught with the bell and to know the safety rules.

*7. SQUIGGLE STORIES (Grades 3-6)

A. Preparation and Materials: Prepare a duplicated sheet similar to the example. The children will need pencils and paper.

*This activity is available in Prevent Volume I of the Spice™ Duplicating Masters.

Example:

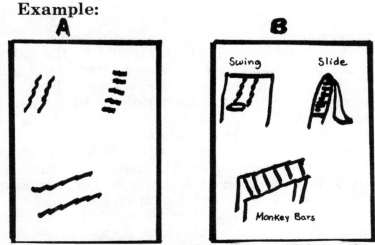

B. Introduction to the Class: Take a few minutes to look at the squiggles on your paper. Can you make a picture of three types of playground equipment from them? Look very hard. You are going to have to add some lines of your own, aren't you? Yes, that is a good idea, Andy. You could make a swing out of those two lines, couldn't you?

When you have found the three types of playground equipment, write a playground safety story about each one. Remember the rules for playground safety.

C. Correlation: Use this technique with a lesson in creative writing.

8. DOG CATCHER (Grades K-4)

A. Preparation and Materials: The game must be played outside or in the gym. No materials are needed.

B. Introduction to the Class: Sometimes, stray dogs on the playground or in our neighborhood can endanger our safety. What would you do Mark, if you saw a stray dog on the playground?

Yes, stay away from him would be the safest, wouldn't it? Did you know some boys and girls do not stay away from stray dogs? They will sometimes try to pull their tails or hurt them in some way. Would you blame a dog if he bit or scratched someone who did this?

Sometimes, stray dogs will bite for no reason. Maybe they have been frightened and they feel as if you might hurt them, too. Do you know what to do if you should be bitten by a dog?

Right, Mary Beth, you should tell your teacher or some other adult right away. They could take you for emergency care and call the police. Dog bites can be very serious.

You should also try to remember what the dog looks like. This will help the police find the dog and its owner.

(Continue discussion according to grade level.)

Now that we have been very serious about stray dogs and you know what you should do, let's play a game. It is a fun game called "Dog Catcher."

C. Directions:

1. Choose someone to be the Dog Catcher.
2. Select a spot to be called the "Dog Pound" and make two boundary lines some distance apart. One will be the starting line. The other will be the finish line.
3. Divide the students into two groups.
4. Each group will decide on a team name. (Example: Group 1, Poodles — Group 2, Collies.)
5. Both groups will stand behind the starting line.

6. The teacher will say, "Go Poodles" and the Poodles will run to the finish line. They will try to make it without being caught by the Dog Catcher.

7. If the Dog Catcher does tag a player, that player goes to the dog pound.

8. The team with the most players left on the finish line after both teams have had a chance to run is the winner.

9. KING PUSHER (Grades K-5)

A. Preparation and Materials: Draw a well defined circle on the ground.

B. Introduction to the Class: There is a time to push and a time not to push. Do you know when not to push each other? Yes, we don't push each other in the classroom or while you are waiting in the lunch line, etc. (Continue discussion according to grade level.)

At the beginning I said there was a time to push as well as a time not to push. Can anyone guess when the time to push might be?

You may push all you like if you are playing a game called "King Pusher."

C. Directions:

1. All boys stand inside the circle. (Girls get a separate turn.)

2. Fold your arms behind you.

3. When I say "Go" try to push each other out of the circle by using shoulders.

4. Anyone who steps outside the circle is out.

5. Anyone who unfolds his arms or falls down is out.

6. The last one left is "King Pusher" of the circle.

10. BUZZ, DASH, BUZZ (Grades K-3)

A. Preparation and Materials: Explain the school "take cover" procedure. Have a practice tornado drill or nuclear attack drill. Show students where to go and how to protect their heads. Ask them to pay particular attention to the sound of the buzzer or bell used to signal this procedure. Play the piano or use a music record for the game.

B. Introduction to the Class: Now, when you hear a series of short blasts or rings on the bell or buzzer, you know what to do. It might be just a drill, but we will always play it safe and follow the school rules.

Can anyone tell me how this type of drill differs from a fire drill? Right, when we have a fire drill we go outside. What does the buzzer sound like if it is a fire drill? Why do you think the procedures are different? (Continue discussion and encourage comparison.)

When you are just learning these drills, it might be easy to forget which buzzer is which. Today, we are going to play a game that will help you remember what the three short buzzers mean. The game is called "Buzz, Dash, Buzz."

C. Directions:

1. Stand in a circle.
2. I will play some music. You may sing, dance or skip around to the music.
3. At some point the music will stop and I will say "Buzz, Dash, Buzz."
4. When you hear this, sit down quick and put your arms over your head the way I showed you for a tornado drill.
5. Anyone who doesn't do this is out of the game.

D. Variation: Play the same type of game after a fire drill. Instead of saying, "Buzz, Dash, Buzz" say "Buzzzzzzzzzzzzz". Again, be sure to point out the different sounds for the two drills.

*11. UP, UP, UMBRELLA (Grades K-3)

A. Preparation and Materials: Prepare a duplicated sheet similar to the example. Additional fill-in sentences could be added for older children. The students could draw and color an umbrella in the top space or this could be used as a good cutting practice activity. For cutting, children will need scissors, paste, crayons and half of a 9x12 inch sheet of construction paper. Allow the children to trace the parts of the umbrella on the folded paper or prepare a traced sheet for each child in advance.

Example:

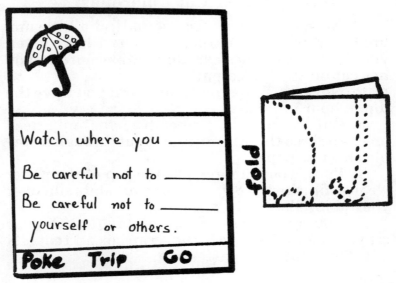

*This activity is available in Prevent Volume I of the **Spice**™ Duplicating Masters.

B. Introduction to the Class: It seems we have had a great deal of rain lately and I notice many of you are bringing umbrellas to school. Did you know umbrellas could cause accidents? Can you think of an accident caused by an umbrella? Yes, Susie got poked yesterday. She was lucky it didn't hit her in the eye. (Continue the discussion as long as needed.)

Today, we are going to talk about umbrella safety. Look at your paper. These sentences are not complete, are they? The missing words are at the bottom of the paper. I will read the sentence and you pick out the right word.

The first one is: Watch where you _____. Can you find the word that goes in that blank? Right, Paul. The word is **go.** Copy this word on the blank space. (Continue with the other two blanks. Discuss the reason for each rule.)

C. Directions for Cut Umbrellas:

1. Now, take your scissors and cut a little umbrella out of the construction paper I have given you. Follow the lines carefully. Make sure you do not cut on the folded part.

2. Next, open up your paper and you have the top to your umbrella.

3. Cut the handle. Remember, you only need one handle so there is no need to cut through a double sheet of paper.

4. Paste your umbrella to the top of the paper we just finished. Now, you have an umbrella over your umbrella safety rules.

5. You may decorate your umbrella with your crayons or you may go to the scrap box and cut bits of colored paper to paste on it.

12. SHOWER POWER (Grades 4-8)

A. Preparation and Materials: Drawing paper, crayons and felt pens. Arrange to post drawings near school shower room. This activity could also be used for lavatory safety.

B. Introduction to the Class: Today, we are going to make a series of "Shower Power" safety posters. We will put them near the shower room door to remind you that there is a need for safety everywhere you go, including the shower.

Have any of you ever heard of shower accidents? I'm sure you have and I'm sure most of you already know the rules for shower room safety, but let's go over them again and list them on the board. For example, what could happen if the soap were left on the floor? Yes, a fall might be the result. (Continue discussion and list safety rules on the chalk board.)

Example:

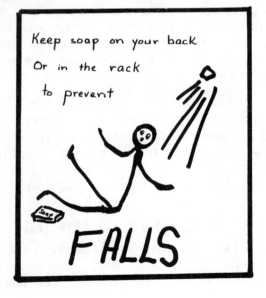

Select a rule (assignments could be made to avoid too many duplications) and illustrate it. You may print the rule on your drawing or you may choose to write a safety slogan to add more spice to your work.

**13. SCHOOL SAFETY VOCABULARY (Grades 4-8)

A. Preparation and Materials: Prepare a duplicated sheet similar to the example. Students will need pencils and dictionaries.

Example:

Ventilation
_____

Monitor
_____

Precaution
_____

Continue in this way using additional words such as apparatus, laboratory, unorganized, organized, hazard, supervisor, spectator and statistics.

B. Introduction to the Class: The words on this paper are words related to school safety. You should be able to understand them. First, look over the list and write the meaning of each word you already know. Then, use your dictionary to find the meaning of each word you do not know.

14. DAILY SAFETY GUIDE (Grades K-8)

A. Preparation and Materials: Use stiff cardboard for back and front cover. Make several pages on the inside. Put together with

**This activity is available in Prevent Volume II of the Spice™ Duplicating Masters.

rings at the top. Print a different school safety rule on each page.

Example:

B. Introduction to the Class: This is our school safety guide. Each morning I will choose someone to come up and turn the page and read the safety rule of the day.

SECTION III: Traveling Safely By Foot, Car, Bus and Air

Never before in history has our society been more mobile. We are a nation of "goers" and "doers." Our means of transportation has become faster and more sophisticated and it promises to become more so. With increased speed and sophistication the possibilities of accidents also increase. Today, even traveling by foot carries increased danger.

Already statistics are proving that there is a tremendous need for safety education in this area. The following games and activities are intended to help your students become more alert to the potential dangers of growing up in a world where motion is the password.

1. SAY IT WITH PICTURES (Grades K-8)

A. Preparation and Materials: Set aside a bulletin board or some other appropriate space for display. Use cut letters or print the caption "Say It With Pictures."

The students will need poster board or construction paper, scissors, paste, magazines, crayons, felt pens or pencils.

Make a list (or encourage students to do so) of words or phrases relating to street safety.

Example:
Jaywalker
Friendly Stranger
Watch Your Step
Bus Safety
Buckle Up
Dangerous Driver
Dangerous Walker
Crash
Danger
etc.

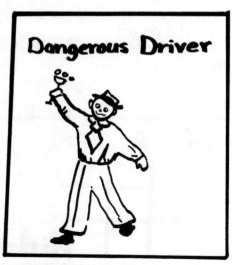

B. Introduction to the Class: It has been said that pictures can say more than a thousand words. Let's try it on the back bulletin board. Select a word or phrase from this list or assign an individual or small group to each idea to prevent duplication. Print the word at the top of your paper. Next, begin looking through magazines for pictures which you think would describe the word. Sometimes, a funny picture can describe the word best and sometimes, you may need to use several parts of pictures to illustrate your idea.

C. Variation: The picture vocabularies could be put together in a class book or if enough time is allowed, the students could make individual books.

*2. BUS GUGGENHEIM (Grades 2-8)

A. Preparation and Materials: Have a school bus driver come in and talk about the rules for bus safety or lead a class discussion. Put the rules on the board.

Prepare a duplicated sheet similar to the example. The students will need pencils. A simple prize for the winner is optional.

Example:

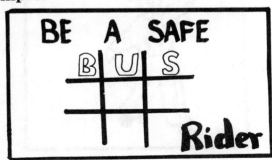

*This activity is available in Prevent Volume I of the **Spice**™ Duplicating Masters.

(Space for writing bus safety rules could be left and filled in by the students for writing practice.)

B. Introduction to the Class: Now that we have discussed bus safety, let's play a game called Bus Guggenheim. Under the word B U S on your paper draw six spaces, two under B, two under U, and two under S. You have five minutes to think of a word to go in each space. You may use any words you like, but the words in the B column must start with B. The U column starts with U and the S column must contain words starting with S.

Example:

B	U	S
baby	umbrella	stop
barnyard	Utah	silly

When you have finished, we will score the papers and discover the winner of the game. Ten points will be scored for each entry selected by no one else in the class, and one point will be given for each entry used by the other players.

Optional: After we find the winner, you may copy the rules for bus safety in the space provided. Use the back of your paper if you need more room.

** **C. Variation:** Safety Guggenheim could be played when other areas of safety are discussed. However, be sure to avoid long words or having too many spaces under each letter as the scoring would take up too much time.

*This activity is available in Prevent Volume I of the **Spice**™ Duplicating Masters.
This activity is available in Prevent Volume II of the **Spice™ Duplicating Masters.

3. STOP, STOP, GO (Grades K-1)

A. Preparation and Materials: None.

B. Introduction to the Class: One way to be safer on the street is to watch the traffic light when we cross the street. We know it is safe to go when the light is _____ . (Let the children answer.) We must stop and wait if the light is _____ .

Today, we are going to think about safety on the street as we play our game. This game is called "Stop, Stop, Go."

C. Directions: "Stop, Stop, Go" is played like "Duck, Duck, Goose," so we must first sit in a circle. Next, I will choose a person to take the first turn. This person will go around the circle tapping each child on the head, saying, "Stop, Stop, Stop," etc. When he says, "Go," and taps a person that person will get up and chase him around the circle. The tapper tries to get back to the other person's place before he is caught.

If he is caught, he must go to "jail" in the middle of the circle. He stays there until someone else is caught. Then that person goes to "jail" and the first person can get back in the game.

When the chase is ended, the child who was tapped "Go" becomes the new tapper and the game continues.

4. INDIVIDUAL TRAFFIC LIGHTS (Grades K-1)

A. Preparation and Materials: Each child will need a milk carton. The half gallon size works well. Be sure to rinse the carton out. Cut an appropriate number of red, yellow and green circles from construction paper. Also, cut strips of black construction paper large enough to cover the entire milk carton. The children will need glue.

Make a sample traffic light to have on display or make a light in stages with them.

B. Introduction to the Class: Did you know that not long ago there were no cars on our streets? People had to watch out for horses, but there were no cars. Today, we have many, many cars and we must be careful when we cross a street. What helps us to cross a street? (Accept policeman and all other appropriate answers.) Yes, traffic lights help us cross when there is no policeman.

The first traffic light was invented by a man named Garrett Morgan. Can you imagine what our streets would look like today with so many cars going in all directions if Mr. Morgan had not invented the traffic light?

Mr. Morgan's traffic light did not look like the ones we have today, but it solved the problem. Boys and girls should learn what the colors on the traffic light stand for. To help you remember you are going to make your very own personal traffic light. You may take it home and teach someone else what the colors mean.

C. Directions:

1. Glue the black strip of paper around your milk carton.

2. Next, glue the circles down the side in the right order. Which one comes first? Right, red is on top. Yellow is in the center . . . etc.

3. Do traffic lights only have lights down one side? No, usually the lights are on all four sides and that is how we will make our lights. Be careful as you turn your carton around to be sure your circles are in the right order.

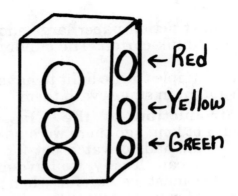

5. SING A SONG OF STREET SAFETY (Grades K-1)

A. Preparation and Materials: None are needed.

B. Introduction to the Class: You all know the song, "Here We Go Round The Mulberry Bush." Today, we are going to change that song and sing it with new words and actions. We will make up some safety verses and some safety actions.

For example, if I sang, "This is the way we cross the street, cross the street, cross the street," what kind of actions could you make up?

Yes, that is a very good idea. We could put our hand to our eyes and look both ways.

Other sample verses:

This is the way we throw away sharp objects . . . (Action: Drop them in a trash barrel. Waste basket could be placed in the circle.)

This is the way we talk to strangers . . . (Action: Shut mouth tight and shake head NO.)

C. Variation: This activity could be used to help children remember safety rules whenever any area of safety has been discussed.

Example: Fire Safety

This is the way we put out fires . . . (Action: Throw dirt or roll in a rug, etc.)

This is the way we report a fire . . . (Action: Dial on telephone or pull fire alarm.)

6. SAFETY HALLOWEEN MASK
(Grades K-3)

A. Preparation and Materials: The children need a large paper bag, newspaper, paste, scissors, paint and brushes. A pan and water are needed for every few children.

B. Introduction to the Class: At Halloween time it is hard to see when you wear a mask. We are going to make funny, but very safe Halloween masks so you can see everywhere you go especially when you cross the streets.

C. Directions:

1. Try on your paper bag to make sure it is much larger than your head. The bag will be a stiff mask when we are done and you want to be able to get it on.

2. Now, let's see where your eyes should go. Wet your fingers a little with your tongue. Now, put your wet fingers on your bag where your eyes should go. Quickly before the marks dry, cut out big, very big eye holes. (If the bag is too long, trim the bottom off.)

3. Fill the bag full of crumpled paper to help it keep its shape.

4. Tear newspaper into strips about two inches wide and eight inches long. (This could be done in advance for very young children.)

Dip the strips in the paste. Paste the strips on the bag. Smooth the rough spots. Cover your bag twice.

5. After the bag has dried, we will paint the mask and cut out the mouth and nose if you want to.

6. You can add yarn hair, paper ears, and a silly nose if you like, but remember this is a safety mask with large, safe eye holes so you can be safe on Halloween.

7. Remember, ordinarily you can see out of the sides of your eyes like this. Let's do it. See how much you can see out of the sides of your eyes. On Halloween you won't be able to see except in front of you. Put your hands around your face like this. Can you see out of the sides now?

So, on Halloween what must you remember to do before you cross the street? Yes, turn your head both ways before you cross because you won't be able to see out of the sides of your eyes.

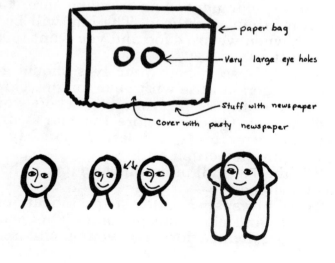

← paper bag

←Very large eye holes

Stuff with newspaper

Cover with pasty newspaper

7. WISE OWL TREAT BAGS (Grades K-4)

A. Preparation and Materials: Have one large, heavy duty grocery bag for each child and one for a bulletin board owl, brown construction paper, one 9x12 inch sheet per child, multi-colored construction paper for feathers, black construction paper for eyes and mouth. Scissors, paste and a felt pen will also be needed.

Introduce the lesson by preparing a bulletin board similar to the example. You will need to make a paper bag owl. Turn bag upside down, stuff and secure at the bottom. Add features and feathers. Put him on a real branch and cut appropriate letters.

Example:

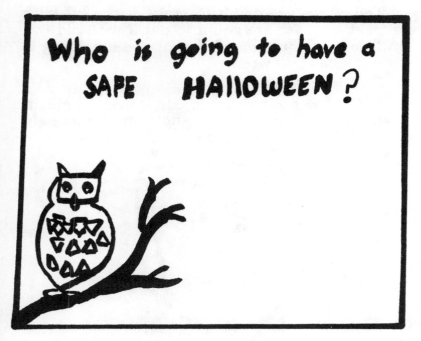

Who is going to have a
SAFE   HAllOWEEN ?

B. Introduction to the Class: Who is going to have a safe Halloween? I'm glad you all raised your hands because safe Halloweens are really the only fun Halloweens.

Trick or treating is fun to do on Halloween and it can be safe if you remember to be as wise as this old owl on our bulletin board.

Mr. Owl advises that you be careful crossing the street and going trick or treating at strange houses. It is very sad, but sometimes people put sharp things like razor blades in treats for boys and girls on Halloween. We don't know why people do mean things like that, but it is safer for you if you only go trick or treating in your neighborhood. (Continue the discussion and gear it to grade level. Some children may have experiences to share.)

Today, we are going to make a special trick or treat bag. We are going to put a wise old owl on it to help you remember that you are going to have a safe Halloween.

C. Directions:

1. Cut, or have children cut, a hand hold in their grocery sack. Cut a hole approximately 2 inches down from the top.

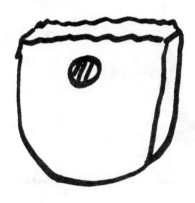

2. Print name at the top of the bag with the felt pen.

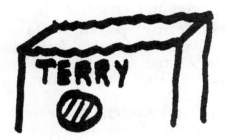

3. Cut owl shape from brown construction paper. Triangles of appropriate size and a circle could be used.

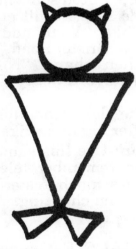

4. Cut black circle eyes and mouth. Paste on head.
5. Cut multi-colored feathers. Small triangles work well. Paste to body.
6. Paste owl to treat bag.

8. ADDRESS CHANT (Grades K-1)

A. Preparation and Materials: Prepare a chart with each child's name on it.

B. Introduction to the Class: Knowing where you live is a good safety idea, isn't it? Can anyone tell me why? Right, Marsha. If you get lost you could tell a policeman where to take you home.

Today, as I take attendance, we are going to play a chanting game which will help you remember your address. Tina Anderson is first on the list so we will start with her. Now, I will chant this sentence to Tina. "Tina, do you know your address?"

She will answer, "Yes, I know my address. It is _____ ." If Tina doesn't know her address yet, she may answer, "I need some help today."

If Tina needs help, ᵀ will chant her address for her like this, "Your address is Twelve, Twenty One East Bristol Road."

Tina will then chant, "Now I know my address. It is Twelve, Twenty One East Bristol Road."

Then, on the day Tina doesn't need help, I'll put a star after her name like this.

C. Variation: Use this same technique later to help children remember telephone numbers. This usually goes much faster as children are used to numbers and chanting.

*9. SEAT BELT SUSIE (Grades K-1)

A. Preparation and Materials: Prepare a duplicated sheet similar to the one shown. The children will need crayons.

*This activity is available in Prevent Volume I of the **Spice**™ Duplicating Masters.

Example:

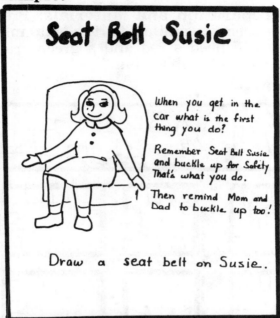

Seat Belt Susie

When you get in the car what is the first thing you do?

Remember Seat Belt Susie and buckle up for Safety That's what you do.

Then remind Mom and Dad to buckle up too!

Draw a seat belt on Susie.

B. Introduction to the Class: This is Seat Belt Susie. She is getting ready to go for a ride in the car with her parents, but she has forgotten to do something very important. Look at the picture and see if you can find out what she forgot.

Yes, she forgot to buckle her seat belt. That is the first thing you do when you get in the car isn't it? Do you remember why? Right, we buckle up for safety. If the car stops fast, you won't hit your head or go through the windshield. (Continue with discussion as time permits.)

Now, let's read what it says about Seat Belt Susie. Then you may color her and don't forget to put a seat belt on her. Use your black crayon to draw a safety belt on her.

*10. WHICH WAY? (Grades K-6)

A. Preparation and Materials: Prepare a duplicated sheet similar to the example. The students will need a red and a green crayon or any other color combination.

Example:

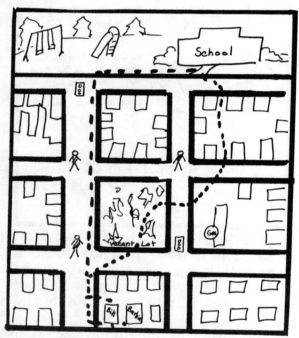

B. Introduction to the Class: Bill and Barbie live next door to each other. They go to the same school, but they do not walk to school the same way. Bill says his way is the fastest, but Barbie says her way is the safe way. Use a green crayon and fill in the route Barbie takes to school. Use a red crayon and trace Bill's way. Which way do you think is the safe way? Why? Which way is not safe? Why?

*This activity is available in Prevent Volume I of the **Spice**™ Duplicating Masters.

11. ROUTES TO SCHOOL (Grades 2-8)

A. Preparation and Materials: Pencils and paper are needed. Crayons are optional. A city or school map would be helpful.

B. Introduction to the Class: Today, I would like you to draw a map of your route to school. Include all of the signs, traffic lights, railroad crossings and places where there is a crossing guard, policeman or safety patrol person. If you find you can't remember all of the safety signs today, you may take notes on your way home this afternoon and finish your map tomorrow.

If you ride the bus, draw a map of the walk you take to the bus stop. Use an arrow to the side of your paper and indicate rules for behavior at the bus stop. Next, draw the route the bus travels and include safety precautions the bus driver observes. Older children may be asked to give details of state laws governing bus safety. They might interview their driver who has been trained to observe these laws.

Example:

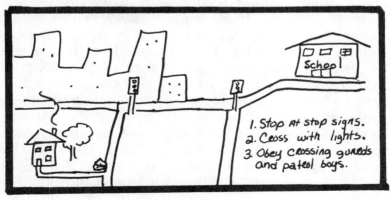

**12. NEVER TAKE (Grades 4-8)

A. Preparation and Materials: Prepare a duplicated sheet similar to the one shown. The students will need pencils.

Example:

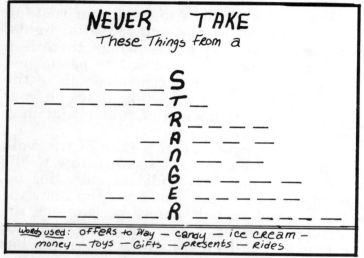

NEVER TAKE
These Things From a

S
T
R
A
N
G
E
R

words used: offers to play — candy — ice cream — money — toys — gifts — presents — rides

B. Introduction to the Class: Probably from the first day you went out to play, your parents warned you about strangers. As you grow older and get busier with other things, you forget some of these basic safety rules about strangers. Today, we are going to do a refresher puzzle which has two purposes. The first one is to remind you again of the rules you learned when you were little and the second is to remind you to keep a close eye on your younger brothers and sisters as well as any little children you may walk to school with or who live in your neighborhood. The words that fit the blanks in this puzzle are at the bottom of the page. See if you can find the right word to fill in the blanks. The letters in STRANGER are clues to help you.

—66—

13. DIRTY NUMBERS (Grades K-3)

A. Preparation and Materials: Young children are very trusting. It is hard for them to believe that evil does exist. As our rising crime rate escalates, the importance of making a child aware of potential threats to his safety cannot be overemphasized.

Read the following example or one of a similar nature to the class. No additional materials are needed.

Example:

One day as Linda was walking home from school a car stopped near her. A man said, "Do you know where Baily Street is?"

"Yes," said Linda. "It is six blocks past our school. You go that way." She pointed in the right direction.

"I've been that way. I couldn't find it," said the man. "Tell you what, I'll give you a dollar if you'll get in the car and show me the way. I'll take you home afterwards."

Linda would have liked a dollar. That was a lot of money and Baily Street wasn't far away. It would only take a minute to show the man, but she remembered what her mother had said about never getting into cars with strangers. So Linda shook her head and said, "No, thank you." Then she started to walk away as fast as she could.

The man drove away slowly. That was when Linda remembered her plan. She turned quickly, stooped down and wrote something in the dirt.

Can you guess what Linda wrote?

B. Directions to the Class: Think about this little story for a minute. What did Linda write? Yes, she wrote the man's license number in the dirt.

Was her plan a good one? Who could she tell about the numbers in the dirt? Why would telling on the man help? Continue with the discussion stressing the fact that a plan could help the police to catch a bad man before he hurts boys and girls.

Now, that we have decided it is wise to have a plan in case we are ever in a dangerous situation, let's practice our plan. We will go outside and practice writing license numbers in the dirt.

What could you use if you can't find a stick quickly?

Yes, your finger.

If there is no dirt, could you write a license number on a cement sidewalk? Right, you could use a stone.

14. SAFETY BIKE HIKE (Grades K-1)

A. Preparation and Materials: The purpose of this activity is two-fold. It helps children to remember bike safety rules when they live in an area where they cross streets with traffic lights and it develops motor control while exercising the large muscles. The materials needed are cardboard or construction paper circles of red, yellow and green.

B. Directions to the Class: Today, we are going on an imaginary bicycle trip. We'll call it a bike hike. Get on your imaginary bike. Hold the handle bars like this. (The children hold on to imaginary handlebars and raise their legs as though pedaling.)

I will lead the way and Joe will be the traffic light. He has a red circle. When he holds that up, we know we must stop. Yellow means caution so we will slow down because red will be coming up soon. The green one means we can go, so Joey, put the green sign up and we'll get started.

Here we go now. Up, up, up a steep hill, down the hill fast and now we go around a curve. Oops, there is the yellow light. Slow down . . . etc.

**15. BIKE DRIVERS I.Q. (Grades 2-8)

A. Preparation and Materials: Students will need pencils and a duplicated sheet similar to the example.

Example:

		TRUE	FALSE
1.	Bike riders are really bike drivers.	____	____
2.	Bike safety habits lead to safe automobile habits.	____	____
3.	Bike drivers have as much protection as car drivers.	____	____
4.	Bike drivers should wear dark clothes at night.	____	____
5.	Bike drivers should have bike brakes checked once in a while.	____	____
6.	Bikes should always be in good repair.	____	____
7.	Bikes are toys.	____	____
8.	Bike drivers need not follow the rules of the road.	____	____
9.	Bike drivers should use hand signals when turning.	____	____

*This activity is available in Prevent Volume I of the **Spice**™ Duplicating Masters.
This activity is available in Prevent Volume II of the **Spice™ Duplicating Masters.

10. Bike drivers are
     part of the flow of
     traffic.   ____   ____

   B. Introduction to the Class: How many
of you are bike owners? Do you ride your bike
or drive it? Some safety experts claim that
bikes are not toys and that people don't ride
them, they drive them.
   Today, we see people of all ages driving regular
bikes as well as motor bikes. With this increase in
bike driving there has been an increase in bike
accidents. Most of these accidents happen to
people between the ages of five and fourteen. Since
all of you fall into this age bracket, I think it would
be a good idea to take time out for a quick Bike
Drivers I.Q. quiz. All of the questions may be
answered True or False.
   If you get all of the answers right, your Bike
Drivers I.Q. is very high and you are a winner. If
your Bike Drivers I.Q. is low, you don't have to tell
us about it, but do try to improve it before your next
bike driving trip.

16. BICYCLE ROUND-UP (Grades 6-8)

   A. Preparation and Materials: Select a
time when the playground is free of other children. Arrange to have someone give bicycle
safety inspections.

   B. Introduction to the Class: If you are a
bicycle owner, it is a safe idea to have your
bicycle checked every so often to see if it needs
any repairs. Faulty bikes could cause accidents.
   Let's plan a bicycle round-up which would
be a lot of fun so boys and girls would want to
come and bring their bikes. We could invite all

of the students in the school who are bike owners. Then, when we have all of the bikes here, we
could have someone give them a good safety
inspection. If your community has a bike licens-
ing ordinance, this may be done at the same
time.

Today, let's start thinking about a safety
bicycle round-up and make some plans.

Suggestions:

1. Safety badges or ribbons could be
made and given to bike owners who pass the
safety check.

2. Bike safety check lists could be made and
the inspector could check off needed repairs.

3. Some students might prepare a bike safety
demonstration.

4. A publicity committee could be formed to
make posters and announcements.

5. Bike races of different kinds could be
planned.

6. Refreshments could be sold to earn money
for a specific project.

17. BIKE CENTER (Grades 2-8)

A. Preparation and Materials: Provide
resource material for an interest center where
students can read all about bikes, bicycling and
bike safety. Provide drawing paper, writing
paper and other appropriate materials for pictures and stories and poems about bikes. Adapt
discussion to grade level.

B. Directions to the Class: I know that all
of you are interested in bike riding. Most boys
and girls are. What kind of bike do you have,
Bill? A ten-speed? Could you explain what a
ten-speed bike is?

What other kinds of bikes are there?

Owning a bike is fun, but bike owners have responsibilities, also. You must keep your bike in good repair. Do any of you know how to make simple repairs? You must also know the rules of riding a bike safely.

During your spare time I would like you to go to the new interest center. It is a bike center where you can learn all you need to know about your bike and bike safety. I have included supplies for writing and drawing. I hope many of you will try some poems, stories and pictures about bike safety, the kinds of bikes, the history of bikes, etc.

18. AIR SAFETY QUIZ (Grades 4-8)

A. Preparation and Materials: Plan a visit to your local airport.

B. Introduction to the Class: Traveling by air sounds exciting, doesn't it? On _____ we are going to visit the airport. Instead of my giving you a quiz when we return, let's prepare an air safety quiz for our guide.

Example:

1. What keeps planes from bumping together in the air?

2. How are planes kept safe in bad weather?

3. How often are planes checked for mechanical problems?

4. How do you know the pilots are well trained and in good condition?

5. Who takes care of passenger safety in the air if the pilot is busy flying the plane?

6. How do passengers know what to do if a plane has to make a crash landing?

7. Are parachutes used in passenger planes?
8. What safety precautions are taken for passenger safety on the ground in the airport?
9. How does skyjacking prevention equipment work?
10. Is air travel as safe as other forms of travel?
11. Are there things passengers can do in the airport and in the air to help keep themselves safe?

**19. A MATTER OF MATH (Grades 6-8)

A. Preparation and Materials: Students who enjoy math will find this a stimulating safety activity. This could be a class project or one for a few selected math buffs. Let them report to the class when they finish.

The students will need current accident statistics. Prepare a duplicated sheet similar to the example.

Example:

Type of Transportation	Miles Traveled in a year	Number of Deaths
Automobiles & Taxies		
Buses		
Ships		
Airplanes		

Figure out the ratio of deaths per passenger mile and see which method of travel is safest.

ANSWER _____
NAME _____

This activity is available in Prevent Volume II of the **Spice™ Duplicating Masters.

B. Introduction to the Class: If someone asked you to tell which method of travel is safest, could you answer? By doing some research and using the math you have learned, you will know and you can be sure your answer is correct.

The safety activity today will help you answer that question.

20. SPACE SAFETY (Grades K-8)

A. Preparation and Materials: Provide pictures and other resource materials on space travel. Students will need drawing paper, crayons or chalk.

B. Introduction to the Class: Not many years ago seven American men were chosen to undergo training to become astronauts. Do you know who they were? Were they the first men in space? (No.) Who was the first man in space? (Russian — Yuri Gagarin — made a single orbit around the earth in spaceship Vostok I in 1961.)

Who was the first American astronaut to make a space flight? (Alan Shepard, May, 1961.)

Can anyone describe a space ship? Look carefully at the space ship at this scene. (Show space scene.) Now, tell us about it in your own words. Can you think what special safety features might be built into this ship? Why would they be needed? Continue the discussion according to grade level. Encourage students to tell all they can about space travel and space safety.

C. Directions: Yes, astronauts must wear those space suits for safety. They would be much more comfortable in regular clothes, wouldn't they? But what would happen if they wore regular shoes?

Today, I would like each of you to take a sheet of drawing paper. Draw a space suit. **Suggestion for Older Students:** Label as many safety features built into the suit as you can.

** 21. TRAVEL SAFETY VOCABULARY (Grades 4-8)

A. Preparation and Materials: Prepare a duplicated sheet similar to the example or put the word list on the chalk board. Students will need dictionaries and pencils.

Example:

Intersection _____

_____

Reflector _____

_____

Caution _____

_____

Hitchhiking _____

_____

Additional words which could be studied are pedestrian, passenger, patrol, stewardess, skyjacker, and altitude.

B. Introduction to the Class: Today, I am giving you a list of words which are all related to safety on the streets, highways or in the air. You should be able to understand them. First look over your paper and write the meaning of the words you already know. Then, use your dictionary to find the meaning of each word you do not know.

**This activity is available in Prevent Volume II of the Spice™ Duplicating Masters.

SECTION IV: Living Safely in the City

A safe city is a happier, more prosperous city. Thus, it is unfortunate that we have no really safe cities today. However, cities do try by laws and regulations to keep their citizens safe. Many of these safety precautions are taken for granted and many are ignored or overlooked. Through the ideas and activities suggested in this section it is hoped that students of today will gain a greater knowledge and understanding of safety precautions in their city.

*1. FRIENDLY FACES (Grades K-3)

A. Preparation and Materials: Prepare a duplicated sheet similar to the example. The children will need pencils and crayons. If possible, have a policeman talk with the class or have some pictures of policemen to show.

Example:

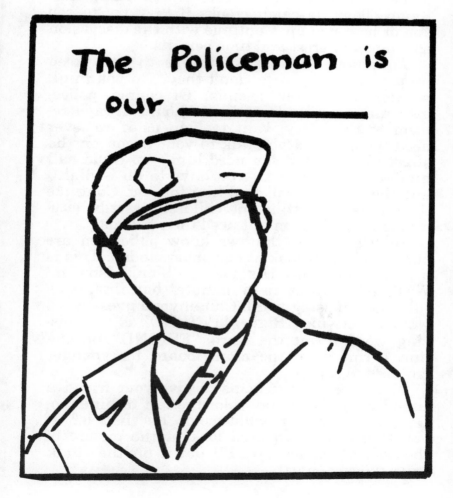

—79—

*This activity is available in Prevent Volume I of the **Spice**™ Duplicating Masters.

B. Introduction to the Class: (Discussion may be geared to a policeman's visit or might go as follows.) A city hires policemen to help keep people safe. This is a picture of a policeman. Can you name some of the ways policemen work to keep you safe? Yes, Shelly, they help you cross busy city streets. And they help you get home if you are lost. Yes, that's right, too, Kevin. They do catch crooks if they try to rob you or beat you up. Continue with the discussion as long as interest and time permits.

Policemen do a lot of things to help keep people in the city safe, don't they? Do you think policemen are your friends? Of course, policemen are our friends and we should always remember that they want to help us if we ever need them. Could you talk to your friend on the street? Yes, and if you need him, you could call him on the phone. All you have to do is dial 0 and the operator will find him for you. Continue the discussion letting the children describe situations where they might need their friends.

All right, now that we know policemen are our friends, let's look at our papers today. This is a city policeman. His face is blank, isn't it? We'll get to that in a minute, but first, let's fill in the missing word. Can anyone guess what word is missing? Right, "FRIEND" is the missing word. Print the word "FRIEND" on the line. (Print it on the chalk board for younger children to copy.)

Now, use your crayons to give your friend a friendly face. You may color the rest of him, too. Do you remember what color his hat is? If you forget, come up and look at the picture of the friendly policeman. I'll put it on the chalk ledge (pocket chart).

*2. FIREMAN'S HAT (Grades K-1)

A. Preparation and Materials: Each child will need a sheet of 12x18 inch construction paper. It can be red or black or whatever color is worn by their local firemen. Draw the basic shape of the hat on the paper. The children will need scissors.

Example:

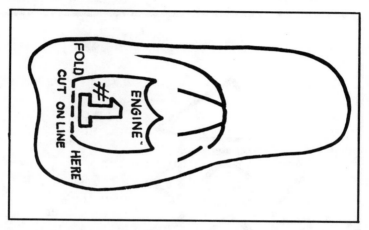

B. Introduction to the Class: Firemen wear a special kind of hat, don't they. Their hats help to protect them when they are fighting fires. It would be fun to have a real fire hat, wouldn't it. We could pretend to be firemen.

We can't have a real fire hat because we aren't real firemen so let's make a pretend fire-hat out of paper. I have traced a design for each of you on this paper. Cut it out and I will help you put it on your head. Then you can go and look at yourself in the mirror and see what your pretend fire hat looks like on you.

The teacher may have to help some children cut the inside holes in the hats.

*This activity is available in Prevent Volume I of the **Spice**™ Duplicating Masters.

A. Preparation and Materials: While this activity reinforces street safety, the primary purpose is to introduce young children to another city helper, the traffic engineer.

A duplicated sheet similar to the example will be needed. The children will need crayons.

Example:

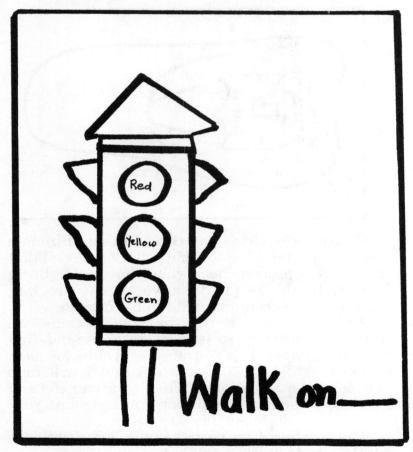

*This activity is available in Prevent Volume I of the **Spice**™ Duplicating Masters.

B. Introduction to the Class: Look at your paper. You know what this is, don't you? Yes, it is a traffic light. They are very important in the city, aren't they? They help traffic to move safely and smoothly and they help people to cross busy, city streets safely. Do you think the city puts a traffic light up just anywhere? No, the city hires a man called a traffic engineer. He makes a study of the traffic problems in the city and he is responsible for placing traffic lights where the need is the greatest. (For example: Discuss a busy corner in the city which the children might be familiar with or talk about a traffic light close to the school.)

Now, let's review the colors on a traffic light. Can you read the color of the top light, Cindy? Yes, it is red. Tell us what red means on a traffic light. Show us a red crayon.

What is the middle color? What does it mean? Show us a yellow crayon. Go on, Buzz, read the bottom color and tell us what it means. Show us a green crayon.

Now, can you fill in the blank space at the bottom of the paper? Let's read it together. WALK ON _____ . Print the word with the right color and then color the traffic light. You may use your black crayon for the pole and box.

When you have finished, I am going to ask if you remember which city helper is responsible for the placement of traffic lights in the city. Can anyone remember right now? Yes, it is our city traffic engineer.

**4. SAFETY ENGINEERS (Grades 4-8)

A. Preparation and Materials: Prepare a duplicated sheet similar to the example.

**This activity is available in Prevent Volume II of the Spice™ Duplicating Masters.

Example:

RESPONSIBILITIES OF A SAFETY ENGINEER

1. Conduct or plan accident prevention programs.
2. Make regular safety inspections.
3. Keep records of any accidents.
4. See that hazards are corrected.
5. Promote safety among management and employees.
6. Participate in safety conferences.
7. Study accident prevention literature.
8. Evaluate safety efforts in order to improve them.

B. Introduction to the Class: Our city has many large factories (change wording to fit your city) where the people work. Did you know that many of these large companies and labor unions employ safety engineers? Do any of you know a safety engineer? Do you have any ideas about what safety engineers do?

The life insurance companies in our area have booklets available about safety. Let's see if our list of ideas about the duties of a safety engineer is similar to theirs.

You can see that many of the safety engineers techniques could apply at home, at play and at school. During the next week I would like you to practice being safety engineers.

You can select one area of concentration for your experiment if you like, home, play, school, or city. Use as many of the techniques of the safety engineer as you can. Explain what you did and we will discuss your evaluation at the end of the week.

5. MR. P. AND MR. F. (Grades K-6)

A. Preparation and Materials: Have available resource material on the policeman and fireman which is appropriate to grade level. Art supplies needed are double sheets of butcher paper or colored paper large enough for a student's body, scissors, crayons or paint, staples and paper clips for hangers. Gear the introduction to grade level. Younger children will need help with tracing and cutting as well as stuffing the figure.

B. Introduction to the Class: Today, we are going to make some paper figures. They will be figures of two kinds of city helpers who work to keep us safe. They both wear special uniforms. Can you guess what two city safety helpers I am talking about? Right, Terry, the policeman is one and the fireman is the other.

Let's divide the class into two groups. Group one will work on Mr. P., our policeman. You may use the resource material in the room to help you dress Mr. P. properly. When you have finished him, see how much you can find out about his job and how he works to keep us safe.

Group two will make Mr. F., our fireman. They will also use the resource material to see how to dress him and find out as much as they can about his job.

When both groups are finished, we will have a sharing time.

C. Directions:

1. Place a double fold of butcher paper on the floor and choose a boy to stretch out on it.

2. Trace around his shape with a crayon and cut out.

3. Color or paint the front and the back.

4. Put both sections back together and staple along one side.

5. Crumple small scraps of paper and stuff figure lightly.

6. Staple other side.

7. Use paper clips to hang.

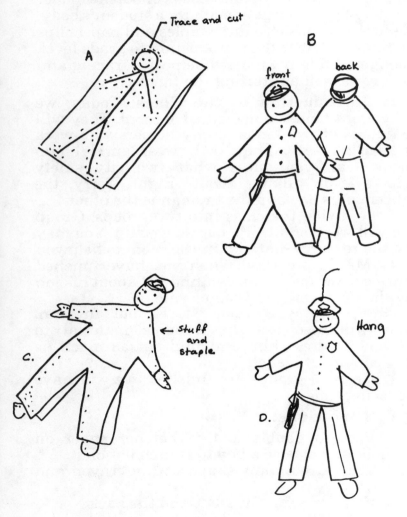

A — Trace and cut

B — front back

C. ← Stuff and staple

D. Hang

D. Correlation: Older children could prepare extensive reports and design a bulletin board display. In the Kindergarten and First Grade the discussion can be correlated with the introduction of the letters P and F.

6. MORE THAN FIRES (Grades K-6)

A. Preparation and Materials: Show a film about a fire department. The students will need pencils and paper.

B. Introduction to the Class: As you saw in the film, firemen do a lot more than put out fires. Did you know that many people believe that is all they do? Is that what you thought before you saw this film? Regardless, you have learned something more about safety in the city after seeing this film, haven't you?

Write this title on your paper:

MORE THAN FIRES

See if you can remember some of the other things firemen do to help keep people safe. List as many services as you can. This can be done through discussion with younger children or they might be asked to draw some of the other things firemen do.

C. Variation: Show other films that can act as springboards for a variety of discussions or notes on safety in the urban areas.

Examples:

(Holt, Rinehart and Winston, Inc.)
1. "The Police Department"
2. "The Trash Problem"

3. "The Post Office"
4. "Public Transportation"
5. "The School"
6. "The Hospital"
7. "The Public Library"
8. "The Shopping Center"

Have children investigate volunteer fire departments. Discuss how these men do their job and what equipment they need to fight fires in rural areas.

7. WHO DUNIT? (Grades 4-8)

A. Preparation and Materials: Resource material on the types, functions, and workings of today's fire extinguishers. The students will need pencils and paper.

B. Introduction to the Class: Can you think of some safety device you see in every school and public building? Yes, Marty, a fire extinguisher is the right answer. Do you know who invented the first fire extinguisher? Do you know how long ago it was invented?

Over a hundred years ago on February 10, 1863, Virginia Alanson Crane was awarded a patent for the invention of the first fire extinguisher. Because of this invention, schools and all public buildings are safer. People who saw the fire extinguisher put out fires knew it would be a good thing to make a law which required one in every public place.

Do you think it would be a good idea to make a law which would require fire extinguishers in private homes and cars? Why?

Today, we are going to divide up into two research groups. Group A will be doing some research on the types, function and workings of today's fire extinguishers. You may use the resource material in the room or library. You may also like to ask a resource person to come and talk to us. You might find a film to show or do an experiment which shows how a fire extinguisher can work. Directions for this may be found in some science books.

Group B will be doing some research also. This group will take a poll of parents and friends. Ask how many have a fire extinguisher in their home? Car? Boat? Camper? Keep track of how many people you ask and find the percentage of people who do have fire extinguishers in their homes and cars. Investigate other places for fire extinguishers not mentioned here.

You may also ask how many feel that a law should be made that would require them to have a fire extinguisher at home and in the car.

8. CITY FIRE PLANS (Grades 3-8)

A. Preparation and Materials: Students will need drawing paper and colored pencils.

B. Introduction to the Class: Do you know where the nearest fire alarm box is located in your neighborhood? Have you noticed where the fire hydrants are located? Continue the discussion according to grade level. You might also discuss how firemen get water to fires when there is no fire hydrant near.

Today, begin drawing a plan of your neighborhood. Use a red pencil to put in the location of all fire alarm boxes. Use a blue pencil to mark the location of all fire hydrants. You may draw simple symbols on your plan and color them with the appropriate color if you wish.

Example:

C. Variation: Discuss what to do in areas where alarm boxes are not used to report fires.

** 9. HAVE YOU EVER? (Grades 4-8)

A. Preparation and Materials: Students will need pencils. Prepare a duplicated sheet similar to the example or write column headings on the chalkboard.

Example:

EXIT	DANGER	NO SMOKING
DO NOT WALK	MEN AT WORK	USE HANDRAIL

B. Introduction to the Class: Have you ever noticed the many safety signs in the city? I'm sure you will recognize most of them on the list I am giving you today. In your spare time see how many words you can find in each safety sign. I will collect the papers and check them before you go home. You will get one point for each word and the person who has the most points will be the winner.

Sample Columns:

EXIT	DANGER	NO SMOKING
1. it	1. an	1. nook
2. tie	2. Dan	2. sin
3. Tex	3. ran	3. go
	4. rang	4. in
	5. anger	5. ink

10. FINDING SAFETY GAPS (Grades 7-8)

A. Preparation and Materials: Students will need resource material regarding their city's safety programs. This might involve personal interviews, city maps giving locations of hospitals, fire departments, etc. Telephone books are helpful in finding out if the city has a blood bank, poison center, civil defense office, etc.

**This activity is available in Prevent Volume II of the Spice™ Duplicating Masters.

B. Introduction to the Class: Every city needs to plan, organize and maintain a vigorous safety education and emergency care program. The goals of such a plan should include ways to correct dangerous conditions that invite accidents and a way to meet emergencies so that accident injuries can be kept to a minimum.

Can you name some safety resources in our city? Yes, Lee, the hospital is an important one. How many hospitals do we have in our city? If the answer is unknown, note that this would be a question that should be answered in their safety survey.

Other Examples of Safety Resources:

Police and Fire Departments
Volunteer rescue squads
Blood banks
Poison control center
Civil defense office
Ambulance service
and others.

Do you feel these services are adequate? Can you think of services we should have but don't?

Today, we are going to begin a survey which involves taking a close look at our city. We want to know if we have any safety gaps. If we do, we will construct a letter to the mayor and tell him about our survey. We can suggest what we feel is needed and give him the reasons we feel it is important.

If, after our investigation, we discover we do have an adequate safety program, I think it would be a good idea to tell the mayor this also.

11. SAFETY SOUNDS (Grades K-8)

A. Preparation and Materials: If possible, make a tape recording of the various safety sounds listed below. If a tape isn't possible, children are usually most adept at producing varieties of sounds with their own voices.

B. Introduction to the Class: Each day the air is filled with safety sounds. These sounds are symbols. Each one means something. Some sounds have carefully defined meanings. For example, what does a fire siren mean? "Yes, Judy, it means get out of the way. There is a fire somewhere."

Some sound symbols have more than one meaning. "Jimmy, can you think of two meanings for a car's horn? Yes, it could mean, get out of the way or it could be saying I'm here to pick you up."

Can you give the meaning or meanings of these safety sounds? Listen very carefully.

Examples:
A policeman's whistle
A squad car's siren
A fire drill gong
A tornado drill's buzz-pause-buzz
Civil defense hum on the radio or T.V.
A truck's horn
A train's toot

**12. APARTMENT SAFETY (Grades 6-8)

A. Preparation and Materials: Prepare a duplicated sheet similar to the example shown.

Example:

Apartment Safety Check List

1. Every floor should have _____ or more

**This activity is available in Prevent Volume II of the Spice™ Duplicating Masters.

enclosed stairways, apart from each other, leading to the street.

2. Each floor should have _____ fire extinguishers and automatic _____ systems.

3. _____ systems that bar intruders are desirable.

4. Each floor should have manual _____ systems which are loud enough to be heard throughout the building.

5. All heating equipment should have been installed to comply with _____ safety regulations.

6. It should be _____ regularly.

7. Hallways and stairways should be kept _____ and rubbish should not be allowed to accumulate.

8. Electrical wiring and appliances in each apartment should be checked _____ and kept in good _____ .

---

condition — hand — fire — two — security — periodically — inspected — clear — sprinkler — alarm

---

B. Introduction to the Class: Many people who live in cities live in apartment buildings. If you live in an apartment or think you might live in one someday, you should know what to look for where safety is concerned.

Today, I am going to give you an apartment safety check list. The answers which fit the blanks are below. Read each item carefully and then use your common sense and see if you can find the right word for each blank.

When you have finished, we will discuss your answers.

Answers:

1 — two, 2 — hand, sprinkler, 3 — security, 4 — alarm, 5 — fire, 6 — inspected, 7 — clear, 8 — periodically, condition.

C. **Variation:** If most of the students live in apartments, they can be asked to check their building against the safety check list. If serious safety problems exist, the fire department or health department might be called to investigate.

13. FIRE ESCAPES (Grades 4-8)

A. **Preparation and Materials:** None.

B. **Introduction to the Class:** In February, 1860, a fire killed twenty people in a New York City tenement. These people were killed because a very important safety precaution was not taken. Can you think what this might have been? Yes, the tenement did not have a fire escape.

This accident was responsible for a safety law in New York which required fire escapes for all tenements.

C. **Questions for Research and Discussion:**

1. What are local laws concerning fire escapes?
2. Do we have fire escapes in our school?
3. What safety precautions do we take in regard to fire at our school?
4. Is there a fire escape in the building where you live?
5. If you live in a single dwelling house, do you have a plan to get out in case of fire?
6. When you are entering a building for the first time, do you notice fire escapes and exits?

**This activity is available in Prevent Volume II of the Spice™ Duplicating Masters.

14. ADDRESS EXPRESS (Grades K-1)

A. Preparation and Materials: Line chairs up in a row to simulate a train or bus.

B. Introduction to the Class: Today, we are going to take a pretend safety trip through the city. Our chairs will be our pretend train. Everybody get on the train. All aboard.

Now, let's start our trip. How does a train sound? Slowly at first, then faster, faster, faster. When we stop, we will blow the whistle. How does a train whistle sound?

Here is our first stop. See the big red trucks. Can anyone guess where we are? Yes, we are at the fire station. How do firemen keep us safe in the city? (Continue in this way and visit one or two safety spots in the city.)

Now, it is time to go home. There are lots of houses in the city, aren't there? Here we are at _____ .Who lives at this address? I'm sure someone on our train does. Right, Linda, this is your house and I'm glad you know your address. When you live in a city, it is especially important for boys and girls to know their address. Do you know why? (Continue in this way until all of the children have identified their addresses and understand the safety value of knowing where they live.)

C. Variation: Reverse the game by allowing children to give you their addresses so that you can "let them off at the right stops."

SECTION V: Living Safely On The Farm

Knowledge of farm safety can benefit every child. The chances of visiting a farm, owning one someday, or just knowing that safety is important regardless of where one is are valid reasons for exploring some of the dangers and pitfalls which might be encountered on a farm.

** 1. CODE-A-DAY (Grades 4-8)

A. Preparation and Materials: Review and reinforce farm safety ideas by placing a daily coded message on the chalkboard. Prepare a duplicated sheet illustrating three simple codes. The children will need pencils and paper.

Example:

1. ADDITION CODE: Add any letter to the beginning and end of each word. RSAFETYT (SAFETY)

2. TURN-AROUND CODE: Spell the word backwards. MRAF YTEFAS (FARM SAFETY)

3. TURN-AROUND ADDITION CODE: A combination of the addition and turn-around codes. Spell word backwards and add any letter to the beginning and end. ZKNIHTY TYTEFASP (THINK SAFETY)

B. Introduction to the Class: Figuring out secret messages is fun and it really isn't hard if you learn the codes. Today, we are going to discover three easy ways to write secret messages.

Look at your paper. The first way is called the Addition Code. This is easy because all you do is add one letter to the beginning of a word and one letter to the end of the word. You may add any letter you choose. Can you figure out the secret word on your paper?

Yes, SAFETY. It could have look like this ASAFETYL. (Demonstrate on the board.) Using this code it still says SAFETY, doesn't it? Remember you may add any letters you want to the beginning and end of each word.

This activity is available in Prevent Volume II of the **Spice™ Duplicating Masters.

The second code is called the Turn-Around Code. In this one the words are spelled backwards. Can you figure out what I wrote?

Right, Jenny. FARM SAFETY is the secret message.

The third code is a combination of the Turn-Around Code and the Addition Code. This one is a little more difficult because you spell the word backwards and add on a letter to each end of it. Let's try writing the word HELP on the board. First, spell it backwards like this PLEH. Now add a letter to each end. It could look like this TPLEHY or maybe this HPLEHY depending on which two letters you decide to add. To figure out what it says, take off the first and last letters and read the word backwards.

Now, can you figure out what I have written in the example on your paper?

Very good, Linda. THINK SAFETY is correct.

Does anyone notice something similar in all three of my examples? Yes, they deal with safety, don't they? And since we have been talking about safety on the farm I am going to choose two people to write a secret safety message about farm safety. In the morning they will put the message on the board and you may decode it in your spare time.

They will use one of the three codes we talked about today. The first thing you must do is determine which code they used. After that the rest should be easy.

Then, the two people will select two more people to write the secret safety message for the next day. We will go on until we have reviewed all of the farm safety ideas we can remember. Some of you may come up with additional safety ideas that weren't covered in our discussion.

If you find you need a suggestion for a secret message, you may talk with me.

Suggestions for Messages:

1. Stay away from farm machinery.
2. Stay away from all power tools unless you are taught how to use them.
3. Keep away from the bull.
4. Mother animals can be dangerous if you make a sudden move toward their babies.
5. When using ladders, be sure they are in good repair and standing on a firm foundation.
6. Heavy tools should not be hung too high.
7. Barns should be well lighted.
8. Make sure old abandoned wells are covered.
9. Watch out for holes in the barn loft.
10. Jumping out of the hay loft can be dangerous.
11. Don't light matches in the barn.
12. Look for wasps nest and keep your distance.
13. Don't play in the tool shed.
14. Ask about any poison plants that might grow nearby.

2. SAFETY SQUIRREL (Grades K-8)

A. Preparation and Materials: Prepare in advance or allow the children to help in preparing a bulletin board similar to the example. Materials needed are background paper, white banner for title, felt pen, opaque projector, coloring book picture of squirrel, brown construction paper, a tagboard nut pattern, tagboard for enlarging squirrel and crayons. Older students could yarn the squirrel for an even more striking effect.

Example:

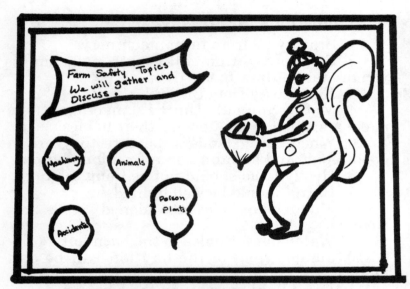

B. Introduction to the Class: Let's get our study of farm safety off to a fine start by making a Safety Squirrel bulletin board. Squirrels gather nuts, so we can cut some brown paper nuts and use them as backing for the titles of topics we will discuss. Our title could be:

Farm Safety Topics We Will
Gather and Discuss

Can you think of some safety topics we can gather and discuss? Yes, we could investigate the types of accidents that happen on a farm. Playing safely in the barn is another good one. Farm animals, machinery and poison plants would also make interesting topics.

C. Directions: Divide the class into teams and make each team responsible for a certain phase of the project.

1. Cover the bulletin board with background paper.

2. Print the title on the banner with a felt pen.

3. Enlarge the picture of the squirrel on a sheet of tagboard.

4. Color or yarn the squirrel.

5. Use tagboard nut pattern and trace several nuts onto brown construction paper. Cut out.

6. Print topic suggestions on white paper and mount on the brown nuts.

D. Variation: Use a coloring book picture of a tractor. Enlarge with an opaque projector and color. Cut a variety of vegetables from construction paper and use these to mount ideas about farm safety. A good title might be:

Harvest of Farm
Safety Tips

*3. MATCHING MOMS (Grades K-3)

A. Preparation and Materials: Make or use a commercially-made picture file of farm mothers and baby animals.

B. Introduction to the Class: As we talk about safety on the farm, we should not forget to mention mother animals. They can be very nervous when their babies are young. Sometimes, they get angry if you try to pick up their babies and if they are angry enough, they can be dangerous. Even a mother chicken can peck hard enough to hurt you if she is angry. Even though it is tempting to touch or pick up and hold baby animals, it is best to keep your distance unless the farmer carefully picks up the baby and lets you hold it.

—103—

*This activity is available in Prevent Volume I of the **Spice**™ Duplicating Masters.

Today, we are going to play a game called "Matching Moms." I have a stack of farm mother animals in this pile of pictures and a stack of baby animals in this pile. Margie, can you match this mom to her baby? If you can, you may choose the next person to play the game. If you don't know right now, I get to choose again.

C. Variation: Older children could be asked to match mother words to baby words. A duplicated sheet would be needed.

Example:

Mare	chick	Cow	gosling
Hen	colt	Sheep	calf
Hog	piglet	Goose	lamb

**4. FARMERS KNOW (Grades 4-8)

A. Preparation and Materials: Prepare a duplicated sheet similar to the example. Students will need pencils.

Example:

1. lulb _____ (bull)
2. yiv noipos _____ (poison ivy)
3. hacinyrem _____ (machinery)
4. msuac nisoop _____ (poison sumac)
5. niaaml iabbse _____ (animal babies)
6. kao sioonp _____ (poison oak)

B. Introduction to the Class: Farmers know that to avoid accidents on the farm there are some things which people must be careful about touching. Do you know what these things are? Unscramble the letters on your paper to find out.

**This activity is available in Prevent Volume II of the Spice™ Duplicating Masters.

5. CHARTING A SAFETY COURSE
(Grades K-8)

A. Preparation and Materials: A large sheet of tagboard or paper to be used for a chart, felt pen for writing on he chart.

Write the following title on the chart:

Things We Want To Find Out
About Safety On The Farm.

B. Introduction to the Class: Have you ever wished you could decide what to study in school and what not to study? This is the title of our next safety unit. What would you like to know about ways to be safe on the farm? You may plan this unit on your own. You decide what we should study and what we should not study. You chart the course and I will help you find the answers.

I will list your questions and comments on this chart. As we find the answers, you may check them off.

Suggestions For Problem Solving:

1. Resource books in the library.
2. Films and filmstrips.
3. Field trips to farms and farm bureaus.
4. Invite a local farmer to speak.
5. Invite the area farm agent to speak or write him a letter.
6. Write to senators and representatives.
7. Collect safety manuals from private business people dealing in farm merchandise.
8. Write organizations such as The National Safety Council and The National Dairy Council.

*6. SPIDER, SPIDER (Grades K-4)

A. Preparation and Materials: Prepare a duplicated sheet similar to the example. The students will need crayons.

Example:

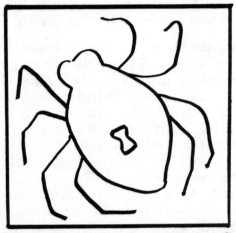

B. Introduction to the Class: Some boys and girls miss out on a lot of fun as well as seeing many interesting things when they visit a farm. They miss out because they are afraid to go in the barn or other farm buildings because they think poison spiders might live there.

Are any of you afraid of spiders?

Did you know all spiders in our country live on insects and that makes them helpful to the farmer. There is only one kind that is harmful to people. The female black widow spider has poison fangs. She can bite, but she is a very shy spider and few people have ever been bitten.

Today, you are going to learn how the black widow spider looks. She is very small and shiny black in color. She has a red spot shaped like an hourglass on her underside.

*This activity is available in Prevent Volume I of the **Spice**™ Duplicating Masters.

Color the spider on your paper like this and remember that all but this one spider are harmless. But, if you should ever see one with a red hourglass on her underside, you're going to know it is a _____ and for safety's sake you are going to get away from her as fast as you can.

7. MAY I, MR. FARMER? (Grades K-4)

A. Preparation and Materials: None.

B. Introduction to the Class: Farmers work very hard to make their farms safe. They build fences to keep their livestock in their fields. What might happen if there were no fences? Right, Mary, the livestock could get out on the road and cause an accident.

Farmers also try to make sure fertilizers and chemicals used on the farm are stored in safe places. Can you think of a reason for this? Yes, Barry, animals and people, too, might be poisoned if these things were not kept in safe places.

Another safety precaution farmers take is to make sure all of their equipment is in good repair. Faulty equipment could very easily cause an accident, couldn't it? Have you heard of any farm accidents caused by faulty equipment?

However, because farms are so big and there is a lot of land, sometimes other people are not as careful as farmers. Sometimes, they go on a farmer's land without asking permission. They leave gates open and are careless in many ways. Some hunters have been known to shoot a farmer's livestock. Campers have carelessly started forest fires and sometimes animals have been hurt because they were frightened by careless trespassers. This is why more and more farmers are posting "NO TRESPASSING" signs on their land. (Continue the discussion allowing the children to relate experiences they know about where the safety of animals and people were endangered by trespassers.)

Today, we are going to play a game which will help you to remember to always ask permission before you go on a farm that is not your own. Remember your safety and the safety of others could depend on this rule for good manners.

C. Directions:

1. All of the children stand on one side of the room.

2. One child is chosen to be the farmer. He gives directions to the others. (Example: Tina, take two giant steps.)

3. Tina must say "May I, Mr. Farmer?" before she takes her steps. If she doesn't, she must go all the way back to the starting line.

4. The child who reaches the farmer first is the winner and becomes the new farmer.

**8. FARM SURVEY (Grades 7-8)

A. Preparation and Materials: Have resource material available on various types of farms, such as almanacs, encyclopedias, etc. The students will need pencils and paper.

B. Introduction to the Class: How many types of farms do you suppose there are in our country today? Let's list as many as we can on the board. You may add to the list later.

**This activity is available in Prevent Volume II of the Spice™ Duplicating Masters.

Suggestions:

Turkey farms
Cattle farms
Tobacco farms
Sheep farms
Tree farms
Horse farms
Dairy farms
Chicken farms
Cattle feeding farms
Truck farms
Sod farms
Wheat and grain farms
Experimental farms

Use the resource material in the room (or library) and see if you can complete the following questions in this farm survey.

Examples:

1. What is the average number of farms in the U.S. today?

2. Are farms becoming larger or smaller? Why?

3. What common safety precautions must be observed on all farms?

4. Would the area of the country affect the type of safety precautions some farmers take? Explain.

5. What types of farm accidents occur most often?

6. One of the functions of the Agriculture Department is called Regulatory. How does this help protect the farmer and the consumer?

9. RURAL MURALS (Grades K-8)

A. Preparation and Materials: A large sheet of butcher paper and art materials will be needed.

B. Introduction to the Class: Today, we are going to begin a rural mural. A mural is a large picture and all of you will get a chance to do some work on it. (Continue explanation of mural according to grade level.)

Before we begin, let's make two lists on the chalkboard. The first list will be the kinds of things we would see in a rural community. The second list will contain all of the safety ideas we want to be sure and include. The rural community we are going to make will be as safe as we can make it.

Examples:

List A
Sky
Ground
Trees
Barns
Silos
Dirt Roads
Railroad tracks
Chicken coops
Fences
Plowed fields
etc.

List B
Railroad crossings will be marked.
Fields where animals graze will be fenced.
Disaster shelters will be available.
Road signs will be placed appropriately on all roads.
Pits and other danger spots will be marked.
etc.

C. Directions: The class will be divided into work teams. Lisa, Gary, Roger and Sue will begin first. They will be in charge of the sky and ground. (Continue assigning areas of work by asking for volunteers and writing names after the items in each list.)

10. COMPARISON REPORTS
(Grades 4-8)

A. Preparation and Materials: Students will need resource material on rural and urban communities, pencils and paper.

B. Introduction to the Class: Use the resource material to make some comparisons with life in the rural areas to life in a city. Pay particular attention to safety. How do safety practices differ? Which environment do you feel would be safest? Explain your answer.

In your report, answer this question. In which type of community would you rather live? Be sure to consider the type of work you think you want to do.

C. Correlation: This activity could be correlated with a social studies unit.

11. MAKING ANIMALS FAT (Grades 7-8)

A. Preparation and Materials: Students will need resource material on cattle feeding, pencils and paper.

B. Introduction to the Class: Farmers have discovered a way to make meat animals fatter, quicker. This enables them to feed cattle cheaper because they can have them ready for market sooner. However, some people feel this method of fattening animals endangers public safety. I would like you to do some research on this subject and then form an opinion of your own.

Copy the following questions in your notebook. These are the ideas you will want to keep in mind as you begin your report.

Sample Research Questions:

1. Find out the name of the drug used to help fatten cattle.

2. Find out why it is now considered unsafe.

3. See if you can discover how farmers feel about this.

4. Ask your local butcher what he thinks.

5. Decide how you feel about it and explain your reasoning.

12. DAIRY FARM SAFETY (Grades K-8)

A. Preparation and Materials: Visit a dairy farm and request that safety be the focal point or have a dairy farmer visit your class and discuss the safety precautions he uses on his farm. Another idea would be to write or call the National Dairy Council representative in your area and request a farm display model or printed material if a model isn't available.

B. Introduction to the Class: Our safety often depends on other people. People who live in the city must especially trust that farmers are following many safety rules. Can you tell us why this is true?

Today, we are going to visit a dairy farm. Remember that we are especially interested in safety. Later, we will make a list of all of the safety precautions dairy farmers must take to make sure our milk and other dairy products are safe for us.

C. Variation: Older students could make a dairy farm model from milk cartons. Attach the list of safety rules to the wall behind the display.

13. RUN, BULL, RUN (Grades K-3)

A. Preparation and Materials: This game could be played inside, but more running room is available if you could arrange to play it outside or in a gym. No materials are needed.

B. Introduction to the Class: When we talk about farm safety, we must never forget to be careful around the animals on a farm. Let's review some of the safety rules we have talked about.

I know a farm game that is fun to play. I will teach you how to play it and each time you play I hope you will remember the farm safety rules, especially the ones about being careful around farm animals.

The name of the game is "Run, Bull, Run". Peter, can you think why this game should remind you to be careful around farm animals? Yes, because the bull is one animal we should all be especially careful around.

C. Directions: Let's all join hands to form a circle. This will be the bull pen. I will choose someone to go in the middle of the circle. He will be the bull and will try to get out of the circle by going over, under or through our linked hands. If the bull gets out of our pen, we will all chase him. The one who catches him will be the bull for the next game.

**14. FARM FUN (Grades 4-8)

A. Preparation and Materials: Prepare a duplicated sheet listing several possibilities for fun on the farm. Allow space for students to make a list of safety rules for each activity.

**This activity is available in Prevent Volume II of the Spice™ Duplicating Masters.

Example:
Swimming

_____

_____

_____

Horseback Riding

_____

_____

_____

Hiking

_____

_____

_____

Hunting

_____

_____

_____

Additional ideas would include: Tree climbing — exploring — pond skating — ball games — fishing — camping.

B. Introduction to the Class: There are many ways you can have fun on a farm. Can you think of some examples?

Doing a thing on the farm can differ from doing the same thing in the city from a safety standpoint. For example, if you go swimming in the city swimming pool you will usually find the life guard on duty and printed safety material around the pool area. You wouldn't find this same protection in a farm pond or lake would you? (Continue discussion encouraging students to make comparisons. They should see that city play is usually much more organized and much is done to insure the safety of participants.)

C. Directions: Your safety paper today has several activities you could enjoy on the farm. Since the farm does not have organized safety rules, I have left space for you to write your own safety rules under each activity. Remember many safety rules will be the same. Example: Always swim with a pal.

SECTION VI: Safety In Play
And On Vacations

Play activities take up a large portion of a child's time. Unfortunately, risks are inevitable and frequently increased when children are lost in the magic of playing. This section has many ideas which will encourage them to think about safety before they become involved in specific play situations. The objective is to prepare them in advance, hoping good safety habits will come to mind as they are required. The teacher's roll is to present the material in such a way that a child is not frightened by rigid play restrictions, but instead realizes that play is more fun if safety rules are remembered and followed.

1. SPLASHY LETTERS (Grades 1-3)

A. Preparation and Materials: Use safety rules as an exercise in printing or cursive writing. The following letter to parents is an example. Print or write material on the chalkboard. The children will need pencils and lined practice paper.

Example:

Dear Mom and Dad,

I like to go swimming. It is fun to play in the water. I know some safety rules for having fun in the water. Would you please help me remember them the next time we go swimming.

They are:

1. Stay in safe areas not too far and not too deep.
2. Before diving in a pool or lake ask, "How deep?"
3. Swim with a friend.
4. Avoid swimming after dark.
5. Don't run around pool decks.
   etc.

B. Introduction to the Class: Because we have been talking about the rules for water safety, I think today would be a good day to write splashy letters. I have put an example on the chalkboard for you to follow. Mike, would you like to read it to the class? Have I forgotten any of the water safety rules? All right, now, as you begin your letter remember to use your very best penmanship (printing).

** 2. GROUND TO AIR FLASH (Grades 4-8)

A. Preparation and Materials: Prepare a duplicated sheet illustrating the Ground to Air Emergency Code.

**This activity is available in Prevent Volume II of the Spice™ Duplicating Masters.

Example:

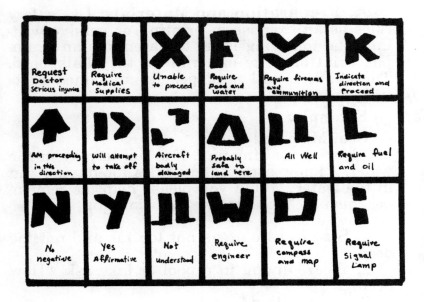

Prepare a set of flash cards. Put the symbol on the front and the meaning on the back.

B. Introduction to the Class: Camping and backpacking vacations are very popular today. Have any of you been on such a vacation? Perhaps you know someone who flies his own plane. Yes, these activities are indeed fun, but they could be dangerous. Have you ever wondered what would happen if you got lost on your camping trip or if you were in a small plane that went down over some remote area?

Chances are someone would report you missing and a rescue plane or helicopter would be sent to search for you. Chances also are that you would have help sooner if you were familiar with the ground to air emergency signal code.

I'm giving you a copy of the code to study. When you have had a chance to go over the symbols, we are going to play a game called Ground to Air Flash.

C. Directions:

1. Divide the class into two teams. They are the rescue pilots. One team could be Red and the other Blue or each team could decide on a special name for their team.

2. The teacher or a student is selected to be the lost camper or downed pilot.

3. The "lost" person flashes the emergency code symbols first to one rescue team and then the other in spell-down fashion.

4. If the pilot knows what the symbol means, he stays standing. If not, he is grounded and must sit down. The other team then gets a chance to decode the message.

5. The game continues until one team is out of pilots or until the pre-announced time limit is up. The team with the most pilots standing is the winner.

* 3. DRESS SID, THE SNOWMOBILER (Grades K-2)

A. Preparation and Materials: Prepare a duplicated sheet which contains "Sid" and several items of clothing. The children will need crayons.

B. Introduction to the Class: Riding on snowmobiles is lots of fun, isn't it? Do you know some of the rules for being safe riders? (Discuss how to hold on, where feet should go, how to get off, etc.) One rule for having more fun and being safer is knowing how to dress. Your parents have no doubt seen to it that you

*This activity is available in Prevent Volume I of the Spice™ Duplicating Masters.

have warm clothes. Do you know why? (Snow-mobile speeds increase the chill factor in very cold weather, making frostbite a possibility.)

Example:

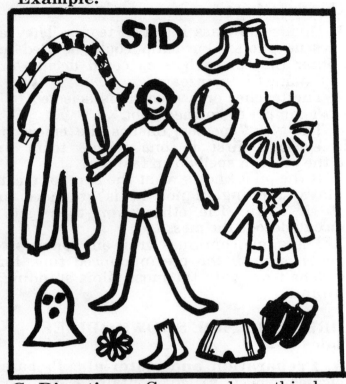

C. Directions: Can you dress this boy for snowmobiling? His name is Sid. Look at the clothes on the paper. Would Sid wear a swimsuit? Of course not. Cross the swimsuit out.

Should he wear a warm snowmobile suit? Yes, color the snowmobile suit.

Keep going. Cross out the things Sid would not want to wear. Color those things which would help Sid prevent frostbite while he is out on his snowmobile.

4. LIGHTNING BASEBALL (Grades 5-8)

A. Preparation and Materials: Children usually encounter lightning while outdoors or on vacations. Resource material on lightning and previous discussions with the class. Prepare a list of questions which can be answered with yes or no.

Example:

1. Does lightning ever strike twice in the same place?
2. Does it always strike the tallest object?
3. Can there be lightning without thunder?
4. Can there be thunder without lightning?
5. Should you stand under a tree in a thunderstorm?
6. Should you swim during a thunderstorm?
7. If you wear rubber soled shoes, are you safe from lightning?
8. Can lightning strike airplanes in flight?
9. Does lightning occur only in thunderstorms?
10. Can lightning start forest fires?
11. Will lightning always kill people if it strikes them?
12. Can lightning rods protect buildings from lightning?

B. Introduction to the Class: Watching lightning is fun. People have watched it for hundreds of years. Aristotle, Lucretius, Descartes and Ben Franklin are just a few of the early lightning watchers. Lightning is a visual display much more dazzling than any of the displays man can put together with tons of fireworks, but lightning can be very dangerous. Knowing about lightning can help us to understand and once we understand danger we can protect ourselves from it.

To help us understand and remember some of the things we have learned about lightning we are going to play a game called "Lightning Baseball". I have prepared a list of questions which can be answered yes or no. We will use these questions to play the game.

C. Directions: Place chairs (or stand) in regular baseball formation. Place an extra chair at each base for batters and runners and also one for the umpire in back of the pitcher. The other team sits on the sidelines.

The first batter takes his place beside the catcher. The pitcher fires a lightning question at the batter who answers it if he can. If he is right, he goes to first base. If he is wrong, he is out of the game. A pinch hitter selected from the children not on the original teams may take his place. Explain that this game has a safety twist. If a player strikes out, he could be injured or dead so he is out of the game. When all of the pinch hitters have been used, the team must play shorthanded.

If the batter doesn't know the answer to the question, he may fire it to the outfield by calling the position. For example, he may say, "Left field". That player must answer the question correctly. If he is wrong, the batter may go to first base and the fielder is out. He must leave the game and a pinch hitter may take his place if one is available.

The umpire permits no prompting or delay. Runs may be scored by moving from base to base. Stealing bases is not allowed.

Play as a regular baseball game for three, five or seven innings. The game may be called due to weather if a team loses three players and there are no pinch hitters to fill in.

D. Variation: This game could be played using any safety subject for questions.

*5. NEVER HIDE HERE (Grades K-3)

A. Preparation and Materials: Prepare a duplicated sheet similar to the example. The children will need pencils.

Example:

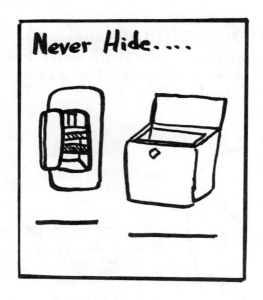

B. Introduction to the Class: Playing Hide 'n' Seek is fun, isn't it? Can you name some safe places to hide, Mark? Those are very good and very safe places, Mark. Can someone else tell us some more safe places to hide?

I'm glad that all of you know safe places to hide. Think for a minute and see if you can think of an unsafe place?

*This activity is available in Prevent Volume I of the **Spice**™ Duplicating Masters.

Our safety paper today shows two unsafe places for boys and girls to hide. Can anyone think of a reason why it would be dangerous to hide in an old refrigerator or freezer? Right, Becky, the door might close and you couldn't get out. There is not very much air inside and that is why it is so very dangerous.

The words at the top of your paper say, "Never Hide . . . " I want you to print the word "Here" on the line under the refrigerator and under the freezer.

*6. GOING DOWNHILL (Grades 2-8)

A. Preparation and Materials: Prepare a duplicated sheet similar to the example. The students will need pencils.

Example:

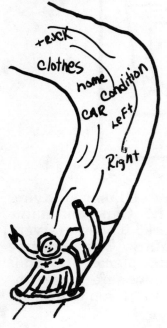

1. See that your sled is in good _____ .

2. Put on plenty of warm _____ .

3. If you go sledding on a busy hill keep to the _____ .

4. Walk back up on the _____ .

5. If you get cold or wet go _____ .

6. When going to or from the hill never hitch a ride on a _____ or a _____ .

*This activity is available in Prevent Volume I of the **Spice**™ Duplicating Masters.

B. Introduction to the Class: Now that winter is here, most of you will want to start going downhill on your sleds. To keep some of you from possibly going downhill in your school work by being absent after a sledding accident, let's discuss some safety rules on sledding. (Accept any ideas for discussion.)

Now, that we have gone over the rules can you complete these sentences? The words are "Going Downhill." Select the best one for each blank.

7. FAIR AND SQUARE SNOWBALL FIGHTING (Grades K-8)

A. Preparation and Materials: The next time a child comes in crying because he or she was hit by a snowball, have a safety lesson on fair and square snowball fighting. Or, if some of your students get in trouble on the playground for throwing snowballs, this also provides an excellent opportunity for discussing the age-old sport of snowballing.

The ruling may be put on the chalkboard as a class project or the students may be asked to write his or her own rules for a fair fight independently.

B. Introduction to the Class: Snowball fighting will always be tempting and fun. However, many schools do not allow it during school hours and the reason is that often boys and girls don't fight fair and children get hurt.

Today seems like a good day to talk about rules for fair snowball fighting. The weather is just right for planning a neighborhood snowball fight this weekend.

Suggestions:

1. All ice balls are outlawed.
2. Snowballs with rocks in them are not allowed.
3. Choose a spot away from houses so windows won't be broken.
4. Don't hit innocent bystanders.
5. Divide up into even teams.
6. Build a snow fort for each team.
7. Any player who doesn't follow the rules is out of the game.

*8. K IS FOR KITE (Grades K-3)

A. Preparation and Materials: Prepare a duplicated sheet with the shape of a kite on it or have the children trace a kite shape on drawing paper. Other materials needed are scissors, crayons, glue or paste, about ten inches of kite string for each child and crepe paper, construction paper or ribbon for kite tails.

B. Introduction to the Class: March is sometimes called the kite flying month. Today, we are going to make some kites and talk about how you would fly a real kite safely.

C. Directions:

1. Color your kite. You may make a design on it if you like.
2. Cut out your kite carefully.
3. Glue or paste a pretty tail on it and punch a hole in the top for your kite string.
4. Now that your kites are finished, let's make a set of safety rules for kite flying. I will write and you tell me what you think are good safety rules. Tell why you think your rule is important to your safety. (Discuss each rule and

*This activity is available in Prevent Volume I of the **Spice**™ Duplicating Masters.

encourage the children to discover any rules they miss.)

Example: Do you think you should use a metal wire for a kite string? Why not?

D. Bulletin Board Idea:

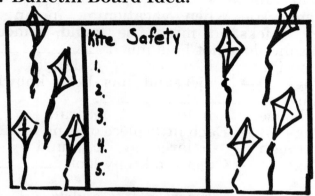

E. Correlation: Introduce the letter K. Use a felt pen to make the letter on each kite and discuss the sound of K.

*
****9. HUNGRY SAND BOOK (Grades K-8)**

A. Preparation and Materials: Use approximately ten sheets of drawing paper for pages. Use the same size colored construction paper for the front and back cover and staple together for a book.

Example:

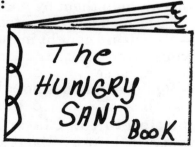

—129—

Print the following statements on each page. Older children might make their own individual books. Statements could be written on the board and copied into the books by the students.

Statements:

Page 1 — When vacationing in an area where quicksand might be found, remember quicksand does not hold much _____ .

a. weight   b. water   c. danger

Page 2 — Quicksand has been known to swallow a _____ .

a. house   b. boat   c. train

Page 3 — Each little piece of sand is _____ .

a. rough   b. large   c. round

Page 4 — Quicksand may look _____ on top.

a. hard   b. wet   c. dry

Page 5 — Most people do not know it is possible to _____ in quicksand.

a. sink   b. float   c. swim

Page 6 — The first thing to remember if you are caught in quicksand is to keep _____ .

a. frightened b. calm   c. moving

Page 7 — Moving their legs makes most people lose their _____ .

a. shoes   b. grip   c. balance

Page 8 — If you see a person caught in quicksand, you can help them by using a _____ .

a. stick   b. rock   c. dog

Page 9 — If you are caught in quicksand, you should keep your arms _____ .

a. out   b. close   c. up

Page 10 — Quicksand does not always _____ .

a. kill   b. sink   c. grab

B. Introduction to the Class: Today, I am going to tell you a little story about some hungry sand. Listen very carefully. When I have finished, I am going to ask you to complete a "Hungry Sand Book" for our classroom safety library.

Hungry sand is another name for quicksand. Quicksand is different from all other sand. A person can sink out of sight without leaving a trace. Once a train, engine and all, was swallowed up by the hungry sand and never seen again.

Do you know what to do if you step in quicksand? Most people do not and that is why we sometimes read of tragic endings to vacations in areas where quicksand is present.

Quicksand is found in areas near water when the water mixes with tiny, round pieces of powdery sand. This makes the sand thick and soupy. On top the sand may look dry. This is why people do not realize the danger when they try to walk on it.

If you step in quicksand, you can get out if you know what to do. First, don't panic. Stay calm and don't move your legs. Moving your legs may cause you to lose your balance and that is when you could go under.

Keep your arms out. Usually by the time the sand has reached your armpits you will have stopped sinking. Then, start a slow swimming motion and move toward firm ground.

If you see someone caught in quicksand, you can help. First, make sure you stay on firm ground. Poke the end of a stick beneath the person's feet. This will allow the air to break the grasp of the sand.

C. Directions: Now that you have heard the story, let's see how well you listened. There is one word missing on each page. As I read the statement, try to remember what you heard in the story about quicksand. Tell me which word should go on the blank line.

Do you remember that I told you not many people know what to do if they are ever caught in quicksand? When we finish our book, you will know and knowing is the best possible way to keep "hungry sand" hungry.

*10. HIKER'S HAZARD (Grades K-8)

A. Preparation and Materials: Prepare a duplicated sheet similar to the example. The students will need scissors and paste.

Example:

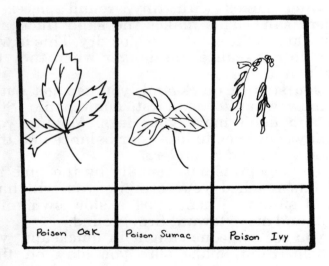

B. Introduction to the Class: Some plants can spoil vacations. They are poison plants and if you touch them or they touch you while hiking or playing in the woods, they usually cause the skin to break out in little blisters that itch and burn.

*This activity is available in Prevent Volume I of the Spice™ Duplicating Masters.

Poison ivy is one of those poison plants. It is a pretty plant with shiny leaves. The leaves are green in spring and summer. In the fall the leaves turn red.

Poison ivy grows along streams, fences and in the woods. It looks a little like a harmless kind of ivy called woodbine. But woodbine has five leaflets and poison ivy has only three.

Poison oak looks a little like poison ivy. It, too, has three leaflets, but they look more like oak leaves.

You can tell poison sumac from regular sumac because it has white berries on it.

Look at your paper. Can you find the poison ivy? Good, Sara, you remembered poison ivy has three leaves.

Now, cut the poison ivy label out and paste it under the picture of poison ivy. Do the same with the labels for poison oak and poison sumac.

NOTE: Older children may be asked to write about an experience they have had with one of the poison plants.

*
**11. SAFETY STICK SKATERS (Grades 1-8)

A. **Preparation and Materials:** A supply of pipe cleaners will be needed for each student. Construction paper, writing paper, pencils, glue and crayons will also be needed. Prepare a duplicated sheet of skating rules. Cut them apart so that you may give each child one of the rules. Also prepare a sample for demonstration.

Suggestions for Skating Rules:

1. Never skate alone. Always have someone with you who could go for help if you should fall through the ice.

*This activity is available in Prevent Volume I of the **Spice**™ Duplicating Masters.
This activity is available in Prevent Volume II of the **Spice™ Duplicating Masters.

2. Obey the signs and be sure the ice is thick enough to skate on.

3. Don't throw anything on the ice. Chewing gum, candy wrappers, bobby pins, sticks, stones, etc., can cause serious falls.

4. Never skate at night unless the ice is lighted.

5. Watch where you are going, especially when skating backwards. Look over your shoulder and watch out for other skaters especially small children.

6. Keep moving on the ice. Don't stop suddenly. Practice figures, spins or jumps only when there is clear ice.

7. When you fall, get up quickly. Another skater might fall over you or cut you with their skates.

8. Don't play tag, crack-the-whip, hockey or other games unless there is plenty of clear ice and you are away from other skaters.

Demonstration Example:

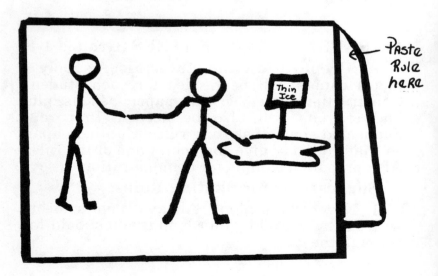

B. Introduction to the Class: Ice skating is fun and it can be safe if you remember a few simple rules. I have the rules here in this box. I'd like each of you to take one and illustrate it with pipe cleaner skaters. I have done one of the rules to show you what I mean.

Can you guess which rule this is before I open the paper?

Yes, Frank. You are right. Never skate alone. Always have someone with you to go for help in case you should accidentally fall through the ice.

C. Directions:

1. Take a rule from the box. Do not look at it, just draw one out and let it be a surprise. Some of you will draw out the same rules, but your illustrations will be different because you are different and your ideas will come out different.

2. Fold your construction paper in half as I did.

3. Use pipe cleaners and illustrate your skating rule.

4. Use your crayons to add details such as facial features.

5. Next, open your paper and paste the rule inside.

6. When you finish, we will play a guessing game. You show your stick illustration and we will try to guess the rule.

* **12. EIGHT FOR BOATING SAFETY (Grades 1-4)**

A. Preparation and Materials: Prepare a duplicated sheet similar to the example. The

*This activity is available in Prevent Volume I of the **Spice**™ Duplicating Masters.

children will need pencils. Discuss the eight rules for boating safety according to grade level.

Example:

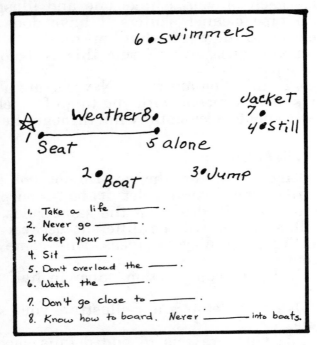

Answers: 1 — jacket, 2 — alone, 3 — seat, 4 — still, 5 — boat, 6 — weather, 7 — swimmers, 8 — jump.

B. Introduction to the Class: Now that we have talked about the eight rules for boating safety, look at your paper. First, follow the eight dots to see what the picture is. Can anyone guess what it might be?

Next, notice there is a word beside each number. That makes eight words altogether. Use these words to fill in the blanks in the eight questions below the picture.

**13. FIND THE MISSING VOWELS (Grades 4-8)

A. Preparation and Materials: Prepare a duplicated sheet similar to the example. Students will need pencils.

Example:

1. R _ d _ _ _ nd T _ l _ v _ s _ _ n.
2. N _ wsp _ p _ rs.
3. W _ _ th _ r b _ r _ _ _ _ .
4. C _ _ _ st G _ _ _ rd st _ t _ _ _ ns.
5. N_t_r_'s w_ _th_r s_gns.

B. Introduction to the Class: Good weather is important to safe boating. There are no rules about the weather that are always true but there are some signs that should always be taken as warnings. If you were out in a boat and you saw lightning in the distance, would you take this as a weather warning? Yes, and you should get to shore as soon as you can.

Thunderclouds are another weather warning. They are a sure sign that bad weather is in the area.

If there is a sudden change in the wind or if a strong wind develops, you know it is time to get off the water. You should never take chances with the weather.

The safe boater learns all he can about the weather before he goes out in his boat. There are five good sources for doing this. Fill in the missing vowels on your paper to find out what they are.

14. FISHING FOR SAFETY (Grades 1-6)

A. Preparation and Materials: A large fish bowl, tub or chalk circle on the floor. Make

This activity is available in Prevent Volume II of the **Spice™ Duplicating Masters.

a fishing pole by attaching a magnet to the end of a yardstick or pointer.

Cut out several paper fish from construction paper. Put enough paper clips on each fish so that they will "bite the hook."

Ask the students to make a list of safety rules for play or vacations. This could be done on the chalkboard as a class project. Put each rule on a fish or have the students do this for writing practice. The next day play the game as a review of safety concepts.

Example:

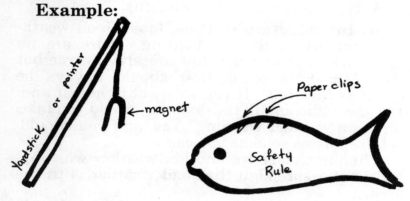

B. Introduction to the Class: The safety rules we have been talking about are now on the fish in the "pond." Today, we are going to play a game with them. This is the way it goes. I will chant:

Example:

A fishing we will go. Donna, catch a fish. Tell us what we should know.

Donna will come to the pond and use the fish pole to catch a fish. When she gets one on the hook, she will read the safety rule on it. If it says, "Always take a compass", Donna gets to keep the fish. If it doesn't, she must let the fish go back in the pond.

When our time is up, the person who has caught the most fish is the winner.

Note: Some safety rules apply to more than one activity so if a child can justify the rule with the activity, he should be allowed to keep his "catch."

Example: The safety rule, "Always carry a compass" could apply to:

hunting

boating

hiking

snowmobiling

or

any other activity where becoming lost might be a possibility.

15. SAFE FEET (Grades K-3)

A. Preparation and Materials: Prepare a bulletin board with white butcher paper. Place a construction paper campfire in the middle and title it similar to the example below. Students will need black construction paper and scissors.

Example:

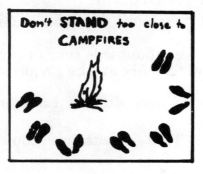

B. Introduction to the Class: Camping trips are a lot of fun, but accidents could spoil them so be safe and tuck some safety rules into your camping suitcase. We are going to use this bulletin board to make a safety rule for you to remember the next time you have a campfire.

Can you read what it says? (Read the title for younger children.) Yes, "Don't stand too close to campfires." Why is this a good safety rule? (Discuss.)

To finish the board, I want you to trace both of your feet onto this black construction paper. Cut them out and put them on the bulletin board around the campfire. Remember not to put them too close to the fire.

16. VIOLENT TOYS (Grades K-8)

A. Preparation and Materials: Discussion should be adapted to grade level.

B. Introduction to the Class: California was the first state to pass a law banning the manufacture and sale of "violent" toys. What are "violent" toys? Can you think of some toys which might be considered "violent?" (Guns, war toys, such as those resembling bombs or hand grenades.)

Questions for Discussion:

1. Why would "violent" toys be considered unsafe?

2. How do you feel about this type of toy?

3. How do you feel about the "violent" toy law?

4. What kinds of toys do you have in your home?

C. Variation: This discussion could lead

into a discussion of toys which are considered unsafe for other reasons, for example, toys with sharp points or loose parts which might come off and be swallowed by young children.

Older students might be asked to do a toy chest safety check. They could check their own toys as well as those belonging to younger brothers and sisters.

Younger students might be asked to draw a picture of a toy they consider to be unsafe. They could then show it and explain why they think it is unsafe.

SECTION VII: First Aid

Training in first aid can be one of the most valuable resources a child can have for his or her safety. While no attempt is made here to give specific and thorough first aid training, it is hoped that children will gain some basic insight and understanding of what to do and what not to do if an accident occurs.

Accident prevention is an important part of first aid education. Thus, the ideas and activities in this section are designed to review preventive measures as well as give general remedial advice.

1. CLASSROOM FIRST AID KIT
(Grades K-8)

A. Preparation and Materials: Have resource materials such as books, manuals, pamphlets, etc., that concern first aid available. Other materials needed would be an appropriate box and materials for covering. A felt pen could be used for making a list of first aid tips for the lid of the box.

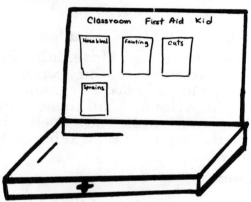

B. Introduction to the Class: We have been talking about the importance of having a first aid kit in the home and in the car. Perhaps we should give some thought to a first aid kit for our classroom.

What kinds of accidents happen in our classroom or on the playground? Can you think of some things that haven't happened, but which might happen? (Continue the discussion and list the suggestions on the chalkboard.)

Some of the accidents you have suggested would require calling a doctor right away, wouldn't they? But there are others, minor accidents, which we could take care of here at school if we make a classroom first aid kit.

Let's divide up into committees. One group will cover the first aid kit. Another will do some research on the types of supplies we should include in our kit. A third group might work on a list of first aid tips which we can include on the lid of the kit.

C. Variation: Invite a doctor or nurse to inspect the completed kit and offer suggestions for improvement.

2. THE BIG QUESTION (Grades 4-8)

A. Preparation and Materials: Prepare a bulletin board similar to the example. Injury topic cards should be folded so students can take them down and write first aid tips on the inside. Large file cards work out well. Research materials could be placed on a table or bookcase near the board.

Example:

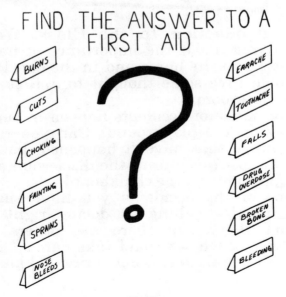

FIND THE ANSWER TO A FIRST AID

BURNS

CUTS

CHOKING

FAINTING

SPRAINS

NOSE BLEEDS

EARACHE

TOOTHACHE

FALLS

DRUG OVERDOSE

BROKEN BONE

BLEEDING

1. Shock
2. Fainting
3. Choking
4. Drug Overdose
5. Frostbite
6. Sunburn
7. Broken Bones
8. Earache
9. Sprains and Dislocations
10. Nosebleed
11. Hiccoughs
12. Bee stings and Insect bites
13. Bumps and Bruises
14. Boils and Pimples
15. Snakebites
16. Burns
17. Dog and Animal bites
18. Puncture wounds
19. Bleeding from Veins
20. Bleeding from Arteries
21. Small injuries
22. Toothache
23. Poisons

B. Introduction to the Class: Some knowledge of first aid can be extremely important to your safety. Some people take complete courses in first aid and that would be a very good idea for you when you are older. For now, let's see how much basic knowledge you can uncover. In your spare time, go back to the bulletin board and take one of the injury cards from it. On each card you will see a certain type of injury listed. Use the research material and find out what basic first aid should be offered. Write your answer on the inside of the card and then sign your name. The person who has his or her name on the most cards will be the winner and will receive a small prize when all of the cards are finished and we have discussed them in class.

3. FIRST AID PIONEER (Grades 4-8)

A. Preparation and Materials: This activity could be done any time during the school year but would be especially appropriate in May as May 21 is the official birthday of the American Red Cross. Resource material on Clara Barton and the Red Cross will be needed. Students will need pencils and paper.

B. Introduction to the Class: All of you are familiar with pioneers throughout history. Can you think who might be a first aid pioneer? The one I am thinking of is a woman. (Allow the students to guess or continue if appropriate.)

On May 21, 1881, Clara Barton founded the first chapter of the American Red Cross in Dansville, New York. She was the first national president until 1904.

I think it is important for you to know something about safety pioneers and I have collected some material on Clara Barton for you to go over.

Examples:

Filmstrip — "Clara Barton, Angel of The Battlefield" (Eye Gate House — 1970). Book — "Clara Barton, Red Cross Pioneer" (Abingdon, 1969).

Look over the material and try to answer the following questions about her and the Red Cross.

Sample Questions:

1. Why did Clara Barton decide to found the

Red Cross?

2. Was it an easy task? Explain.

3. How is the Red Cross concerned with safety? List as many of their specific programs as you can. Examples: disaster relief — first aid courses — water safety instruction — blood banks, etc.

**4. FIRST AID VOCABULARY (Grades 4-8)

A. Preparation and Materials: Prepare a duplicated sheet similar to the example. Students will need dictionaries and pencils.

Example:

Fracture
_____

Stimulant
_____

Sprain
_____

Dislocation
_____

Continue in this way with words, such as suffocation, artificial respiration, internally, sterile, compress, tourniquet, and tetanus.

B. Introduction to the Class: The words on this list are all words which are related to first aid. You should be able to understand them. First, look over your paper and write the meaning of each word you already know. Then use your dictionary to find the meaning of each word you do not know.

**This activity is available in Prevent Volume II of the Spice™ Duplicating Masters.

5. MITTEN-MITTEN (Grades K-3)

A. Preparation and Materials: The children will need drawing paper, crayons and scissors.

B. Introduction to the Class: How do you keep your hands warm when you go out to play in the wintertime, John? Yes, you wear your mittens. Mittens keep your hands warm and safe from frostbite. Does anyone know what frostbite is? Well, it happens when a part of your body freezes. This can be very dangerous. A doctor should be called if a part of your body freezes. You should never rub snow on a place that is frostbitten, nor should you break any blisters that might form. You could press your hand on the spot, but don't rub. You could also use warm water or warm wool blankets to help until you can get to a doctor. But the best thing is not to get frostbite in the first place. Warm mittens can help keep your hands and fingers from freezing, can't they?

Let's pretend for a minute that Lisa forgot her mittens and she has to be outside for a very long time. The wind is blowing and that makes it feel much colder. There are some things she could do to prevent frostbite. Can you guess what they might be?

Right, Bobby, she could put her hands in her pockets. She could also put them on her face or some other warm part of her body. She could clap her hands like this to keep the blood moving or do them like this. (Demonstrate flexing the fingers.) But the best way to prevent frostbite is to remember to wear your mittens.

Today, we are going to make some paper mittens to help you remember to always wear your mittens in the wintertime.

C. Directions:

1. Trace around the shape of your hand. (Demonstrate.)

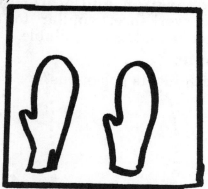

2. Remember to do it two times. You have two hands and you need two mittens.

3. Now, color your mittens. You may make them with a pretty pattern, but be sure to make it the same way on the other mitten so they will match.

4. Cut out your mittens and I'll staple them together for you.

Bulletin Board Idea:

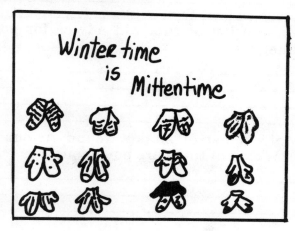

6. SNAKES FOR SAFETY'S SAKE (Grades 4-8)

A. Preparation and Materials: Prepare a duplicated worksheet similar to the example. Have resource material available.

Example:

1. Which bite is poisonous?

2. There are four poisonous snakes in the United States. Name them.

    a. _____

    b. _____

    c. _____

    d. _____

3. Name some things you can do to prevent snakebite.

_____

_____

4. Make a list of first aid advice for poisonous snakebites.

_____

_____

_____

_____

5. Make a list of snakes found in our community. Which of them are poisonous?

_____

_____

_____

This activity is available in Prevent Volume II of the **Spice™ Duplicating Masters.

6. Name poisonous snakes found in other countries.

Snake   Native to What Country

_____

_____

_____

_____

B. Introduction to the Class: For years people have been both frightened and fascinated by snakes. Unfortunately, many people have also been killed by snakes. Some of these people might have lived if they or someone with them had known some snake first aid. Today, we are going to concentrate on knowing enough about Snakes for Safety's Sake.

I'm going to give each of you a worksheet with some questions you can answer. You may use the resource materials here at school or you may wish to look up the answers at home.

Pay particular attention to the questions regarding prevention and first aid. What should you do if you are accidentally bitten by a poisonous snake? What should you do if someone you are with is bitten and what are some things you might do to prevent being bitten? We will be discussing your answers in class.

C. Variations: Prepare a class booklet on snakes. Find pictures of snakes and classify them as poisonous or non-poisonous. Draw pictures of snakes. Clip newspaper articles involving snakebite accidents.

* 7. RUB-A-DUB-DUB (Grades K-6)

A. Preparation and Materials: Prepare a duplicated sheet similar to the example. Students will need pencils.

*This activity is available in Prevent Volume I of the **Spice**™ Duplicating Masters.

Example:

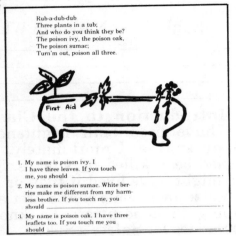

Rub-a-dub-dub
Three plants in a tub;
And who do you think they be?
The poison ivy, the poison oak,
The poison sumac;
Turn'm out, poison all three.

First Aid

1. My name is poison ivy. I
   have three leaves. If you touch
   me, you should _____

2. My name is poison sumac. White berries make me different from my harmless brother. If you touch me, you
   should _____

3. My name is poison oak. I have three
   leaflets too. If you touch me you
   should _____

B. Introduction to the Class: Today, we are going to work some riddles together and see if you can figure out what to do if you should accidentally step in a patch of poison plants.

First, look at your paper. Kate, will you read the verse at the top? Thank you. There is a clue in the verse to tell you what to do if you touch poison plants.

Bill, read the first riddle. Can you find the answer? Very good, Rub-a-dub-dub is the answer and scrubbing yourself good is about the only thing you can do. Use a strong soap if you can. This may help prevent the blisters and itching. If blisters do develop, be careful not to break them. It can spread.

Before we go on to riddle two, fill in the blank line after riddle one. The answer is Rub-a-dub-dub.

(Continue with the other two riddles in the same way. The children will enjoy discovering that the answer is the same for all three.)

Now, write the key to first aid treatment of poison plant exposure on the tub. What's the answer again? Right, it is Rub-a-dub-dub.

After doing this lesson, I don't think any of you will be in doubt about what to do if you touch poison plants, do you?

** 8. MR. BONES (Grades 4-8)

A. Preparation and Materials: Have first aid resource material, pencils, colored pens available. Prepare a duplicated sheet similar to the example or ask the students to draw or trace their own skeleton on white paper.

Example:

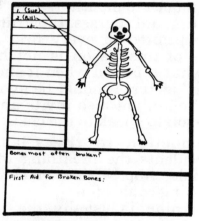

B. Introduction to the Class: How many of you have ever had a broken bone? Do you know someone who has had a broken bone? I'm sure you all do and today, we are going to do a survey to see if we can answer the question: Which bones are most often broken? I would like you to also do some research and find out what first aid should be given if you or someone you know should break a bone.

—155—

Look at your paper. This is Mr. Bones. List the names of people you know who have broken a bone down the side of the paper. Use a colored pen and draw a line to the bone which they broke. When you finish, you should be able to answer the first question at the bottom of the paper.

Then, use the resource material in the room and write the first aid to be given for broken bones.

9. RESCUE BREATHING (Grades 4-8)

A. Preparation and Materials: The procedure for mouth-to-mouth rescue breathing is basic in all first aid courses. Illustrations for how to do it are printed in every first aid manual. The purpose of this lesson is not how to do it, but rather what it is and when it should be used. The "how-to" pictures should be available in the classroom. You might also invite an appropriate resource person to speak to the class.

B. Introduction to the Class: In some types of accidents the breathing of the person involved could stop. Think of some accidents where breathing could stop.

Yes, drowning is usually the first type of accident that comes to mind. Can you think of others?

Suggestions:
1. Drowning
2. Electric shock
3. Choking
4. Overdose of medicine
5. Carbon monoxide poisoning

When the breathing stops or is very faint, mouth-to-mouth rescue breathing could save the person's life. Can anyone give us an example? Perhaps someone you know has saved a life this way.

These pictures show how mouth-to-mouth rescue breathing is done. You will be given proper instructions in how to do this when you take a course in first aid. (Or, I have invited _____ to demonstrate the procedure.)

Watch the newspaper and clip any articles which say a life was saved by someone using mouth-to-mouth rescue breathing. Bring them to school and we will discuss them in class.

10. KNOW A KNOT (Grades 4-8)

A. Preparation and Materials: Follow the illustration below and practice making a square knot so that you may demonstrate to the class. Have scarfs or pieces of old sheets available for practice.

Example:

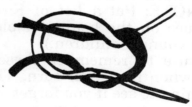

B. Introduction to the Class: Learning to tie a square knot has many uses, particularly in first aid. This type of knot is easy to tie and it doesn't slip. Knowing how to tie this simple knot might save your life someday. Can you think how?

Examples:

1. Tying sheets together to make an emergency fire escape.

2. Tying two ropes together to make difficult rescues.

3. Make first aid bandages longer by tying two together.

I am giving each of you two pieces of this old sheet so that you may practice making a square knot. (Illustrate procedure.)

*11. TELEPHONE TIME (Grades K-8)

A. Preparation and Materials: Pretend there is a telephone in the room or use a real phone (disconnected) or a toy phone.

B. Introduction to the Class: Sometimes the best first aid you can give an injured person is to get help fast. Knowing how to use the telephone can be valuable first aid knowledge.

Today, we are going to invent some accident situations and you will take turns getting help. We will want to know who you are calling and why. (NOTE: Put a list of First Aid telephone techniques on the board for older children. Explain to younger children.)

Be sure to remember these telephone techniques when it is your turn. The rest of us will be listening to see if you forget anything.

First Aid Telephone Techniques:

1. Try not to panic.
2. Remember to speak clearly.
3. Tell who is calling.
4. Tell what has happened.
5. Give your address or location.

Examples of Situations:

1. A child has fallen into a construction hole or some other tight place. You cannot reach him.

*This activity is available in Prevent Volume I of the Spice™ Duplicating Masters.

2. There is a fire in an apartment house. You see someone on the roof, but there is no way you can personally help him.

3. You find someone on the floor. He is alive, but you don't know what is wrong and he can't tell you. It may be a heart attack, overdose of drugs, poison, or a serious fall.

4. You see a person pulled from a swimming pool. Someone has started mouth-to-mouth resuscitation. They tell you to call for help.

5. A person is stung by a bee. He is allergic to bee stings. He passes out.

6. You see someone who is bleeding severely. No one knows what to do. Take charge. Show someone how to hold a pressure bandage over the wound and then call for help.

12. RED HOT TOSS (Grades K-3)

A. Preparation and Materials: A ball, a pan of cold water and a towel are needed.

B. Introduction to the Class: What should you do if you get a very bad burn? Yes, you will need to see a doctor. Do you need to go to a doctor everytime you burn yourself? No, sometimes you get just a little burn and you can make it feel better with some simple first aid. (Continue discussion helping children to see that cold water is acceptable first aid for minor burns.)

We are going to play a game today. It will be fun and it will help you remember what to do if you should get a little burn. We will pretend that this ball is red hot. It will burn you if you are caught holding it.

The cold water in this pan will be the first aid station.

C. Directions: Stand in a circle. Larry can be the caller. He will stand with his back to you. When he says "Go", start passing the ball around the circle as fast as you can without dropping it. When Larry says "Stop", the person who has the ball gets burned. He must then run to the pan and soak his hand in the cold water until someone else is burned. He then dries his hand and sits down. He is out of the game. Remember accidents can stop you from having fun and that is why you should avoid them if possible.

The idea of this game is not to get burned, but each time Larry says "Stop", someone will be burned. The last person in the circle will be the winner. He will be the caller for the next game.

13. WHAT TO DO WHEN (Grades 5-8)

A. Preparation and Materials: Prepare a duplicated sheet listing several first aid treatments. Under this make a list of accidents. Students will need pencils.

Examples:

1. Remove victim to fresh air and apply rescue breathing. _____

2. Induce vomiting by finger gagging after a generous drink of tepid water. _____

3. Lie down in the grass and roll. _____

4. Apply cold water. _____

5. Apply pressure bandage. _____

6. Keep victim lying down. Prevent loss of body heat and give encouragement. _____

Shock — ingested poisoning (non-corrosive) drowning — minor burns -- burning clothes — carbon monoxide poisoning — severe bleeding.

**This activity is available in Prevent Volume II of the Spice™ Duplicating Masters.

Answers:

1. Carbon monoxide poisoning and drowning
2. Ingested poisoning (non-corrosive)
3. Burning clothes
4. Minor burns
5. Severe bleeding
6. Shock

B. Introduction to the Class: We have been discussing the many types of first aid that can be given in a variety of accidents. We have learned that a certain type of accident requires a certain type of first aid, haven't we?

Remembering What To Do When can be vitally important. On your paper you will see several types of first aid treatment. Read each carefully. Then, see if you can match the accidents at the bottom of the paper to the proper first aid treatment.

*14. KNOW ABOUT NOSES (Grades K-3)

A. Preparation and Materials: Prepare a duplicated sheet similar to the example.

Example:

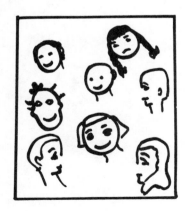

*This activity is available in Prevent Volume I of the Spice™ Duplicating Masters.

B. Introduction to the Class: Nosebleeds are scary but usually not very serious. They can happen if you accidentally get hit in the nose or sometimes for other reasons like a bad cold or an allergy. Anything that might cause the little blood vessels in the lining of your nose to break can cause a nosebleed.

First aid for nosebleeds is usually very simple. Sit with your head slightly tilted back. Breathe through your mouth and gently press your nostrils together at the tip of your nose like this. (Demonstrate.) Can you do that? Sure you can. (Give students a chance to practice.)

If you hold your nose this way for five or six minutes, the bleeding usually stops. If it doesn't, a doctor should be called.

I have a funny paper for you to do today. It will help you to remember the first aid treatment for nosebleeds. Look carefully at your paper. What is missing from each face? Yes, the noses are missing. You add the noses. You can make them long, short, fat, skinny or anyway you like. When you are finished, I am going to ask you if you remember the first aid treatment for nosebleed.

SECTION VIII: Safety Through Civil Defense

Civil defense could be thought of as disaster preparedness. Disaster could occur anytime and anyplace. It may be a peacetime disaster, such as a flood, fire, hurricane, blizzard, or earthquake; or it could be an enemy nuclear attack. In any case lives could be saved if people are prepared for emergencies and know what action to take.

The following activities are intended to help children become aware of emergency action and facilities. As they become aware and begin to understand the nature of danger, it is hoped that they can learn to control it or at least learn to live with it.

** 1. WHAT IS CIVIL DEFENSE?
(Grades 6-8)

A. Preparation and Materials: Write to the Department of Defense, Office of Civil Defense, Washington, D.C., and request a copy or copies for your class of the citizen's handbook on emergency preparedness. Use this handbook as resource material and prepare a duplicated sheet of multiple choice questions and answers. Students will need pencils.

Example:

1. Civil Defense means:
   a. A family plan for protection during nuclear attack.
   b. A system organized by local government in cooperation with the Federal government to reduce the loss of life in a major emergency.
   c. A term used to describe the activities of the Red Cross after a disaster, such as a tornado, flood, or fire.
2. The attack warning signal is:
   a. 3 to 5 minutes of wavering sound or a series of short blasts on whistles or horns.

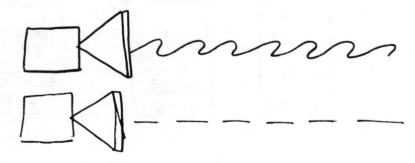

   b. One continuous blast.

**This activity is available in Prevent Volume II of the Spice™ Duplicating Masters.

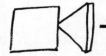

c. One short and one long blast on whistles or horns every ten minutes.

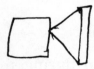

3. The heart of the civil defense system is:
   a. U.S. Air Force antimissile bases prepared to attack if we are attacked.
   b. Money provided by the national government to operate an effective spy system to warn of impending disaster.
   c. The fallout shelter.
4. Public fallout shelters are marked like:

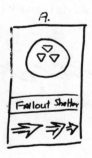

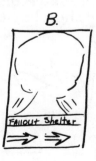

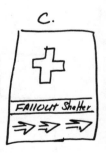

5. Civil defense is an emergency action plan to:
   a. Make people feel safe even though it is a fact no one can survive a nuclear attack or other disasters.
   b. To save lives in the event of a nuclear attack or other disasters.
   c. Mobilize the citizens of our country to fight the enemy.

B. Introduction to the Class: All of you have probably heard the term "civil defense". Do you know what it means in terms of your safety or the safety of the country? Answer the questions on the sheet to find out how much you know about it. When you have finished, we will discuss your answers and make plans for finding out more about civil defense in our area.

C. Variation: Give each student a copy of the citizen's handbook or other resource material. Have each one write a clear question and answer. Collect these and divide the class into teams. Have a classroom quiz using the student made questions and answers.

2. DESIGNING A DISASTER SHELTER (Grades 6-8)

A. Preparation and Materials: Resource materials concerning the factors involved in designing an adequate disaster shelter and a previous discussion of the material and the reasons for need involved. Prepare a duplicating master or wall chart containing some basic facts for construction.

Example:

1. About 12 square feet is estimated to be

essential for one person.

2. Exhaust pipe and air intake pipe are necessary.

3. Storage units for a two week supply of food and provisions.

The children will need drawing paper and pencils.

B. Introduction to the Class: We have been talking about disaster shelters and today, let's try our hand at designing one for our family. (The teacher may want to show a sample design for his or her family.)

I have placed some of the basic facts for construction and design on this chart. They will help you remember what is needed in your design.

Will every design in the class be exactly alike? Why not? Yes, item number one on the chart tells us we need about 12 square feet for one person and some families are larger than others.

C. Correlation: This activity could be correlated with math or a class in scale drawing.

**3. FALLOUT FALLACIES (Grades 7-8)

A. Preparation and Materials: Have resource material on fallout from textbooks, library materials, magazines, government publications, etc., available. Prepare a duplicated sheet of several paragraphs. Each paragraph should contain one fallacy. Leave space so student can write reason they believe what they have underlined is a fallacy.

Example: (Answers are included.)

This activity is available in Prevent Volume II of the **Spice™ Duplicating Masters.

1. In dangerously affected areas the fallout particles would look like grains of sand or salt. The rays given off by these particles can be tasted, smelled and felt.

Reason: Rays cannot be tasted, felt or smelled. Special instruments would be needed to detect the rays and measure intensity.

2. Fallout would be widespread after a nuclear attack. The range of a nuclear explosion is so tremendous no area of the U.S. could be sure of not getting fallout, and it is probable that some fallout particles would be deposited on most of the country.

Reason: The distribution of fallout particles would depend on wind currents, weather conditions and other factors, not the range of the nuclear explosion.

B. Introduction to the Class: Nuclear attack, radiation damage and fallout are frightening words. We all hope we never have to face such a terrifying disaster. However, we must be realistic and consider that we do live in a world where such a thing could happen.

Some people think there would be no hope if we should become victims of a nuclear attack. This is a fallacy. There are other fallacies we should explore for our general knowledge.

C. Directions: I am giving you a paper containing several paragraphs on fallout. In each paragraph there is one fallacy. Let's divide the class into two groups. Each group will work as a team and try to find the fallacy. Your team will get one point if you underline it correctly. You will get two additional points if you can explain why what you underlined is a fallacy. You may use the resource material in the room.

*4. THE ARROW POINTS THE WAY (Grades K-4)

A. Preparation and Materials: Prepare duplicated sheets similar to fallout shelter signs but leave off the top symbol. Cut or have children cut one black circle and three triangles each from construction paper. They will also need paste.

Example:

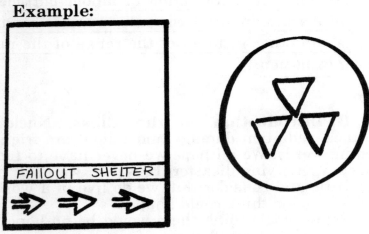

B. Introduction to the Class: If you should hear the disaster warning signal, you know right away that something bad is about to happen very soon. It might be that a tornado is on the way or even that a bomb might be dropped. Regardless of what it is, you know that you must quickly find shelter. We have talked about what

—170—

to do if you are at home or school, but what if you were downtown shopping? Where could you go?

You would look for a civil defense shelter sign which looks something like this. Usually, these signs are on big buildings like hospitals, churches, or big department stores. The arrows on the signs tell you which way to go.

Today, we are going to cut and paste posters which will help you remember what the signs look like. The next time you are out shopping with your parents, see if you can find a shelter sign. If you find one, you will know that is a building where you can go if you hear the disaster warning signal.

See how many fallout shelter signs you can find. Ask your parents to help you.

C. Correlation: This would be a good activity to correlate with a math lesson on learning shapes.

****5. SURVIVAL COOKBOOKS**
(Grades 4-8)

A. Preparation and Materials: Prepare a duplicated sheet containing a list of suggested food to be stored in disaster shelters or to be kept on hand at home for emergencies.

Students will need pencils, paper and resource material on nutrition.

Duplicating equipment for reproducing the menus in cookbook form will also be required.

B. Introduction to the Class: Today, I am giving you a list of foods suggested by the De-

**This activity is available in Prevent Volume II of the Spice™ Duplicating Masters.

partment of Civil Defense as appropriate for keeping in disaster shelters. I would like each of you to study the list and do some research on nutrition. Then, see if you can plan three survival menus. Try to do one for breakfast, one for lunch, and one for dinner.

Because of the food limitations some of your menus will be the same. We will select as many different ideas as possible and put them together in a Survival Cookbook. Then you will each have a copy to take home.

C. Variation: Select one menu. Ask the students to bring in needed items from home. Allow them to prepare and serve it to the class. If a kitchen is not available, help students to understand that this might be the situation if a disaster should occur, so a menu which requires no cooking or refrigeration must be selected for the experiment.

6. SURVIVAL GAMES (Grades 4-8)

A. Preparation and Materials: Provide, or ask students to provide, a box such as the kind stockings come in or a stationery box. Shoe boxes would be another possibility. Some community stores will often give a generous supply of boxes to teachers upon request. Classroom art supplies should be available and students should be encouraged to provide any additional materials they might select.

B. Introduction to the Class: Since people must plan to remain in a disaster shelter anywhere from a few hours to several days, it is a good idea to have books and recreational activities on hand. Today, I am going to make an assignment which will take some creative thinking on your part. I would like you to invent a survival game.

Here are some boxes you may use to store your game in. You may make any type of game that appeals to you or you may wish to think about a game that would appeal to a younger brother or sister. You might even make a game that your whole family could play.

You may use cards or dice or any other materials which you could make.

When everyone is finished (time limit may be given), we will have all of the games on display. You will each get a turn to tell how your game is played.

7. MAJOR DISASTERS (Grades 6-8)

A. Preparation and Materials: Have resource materials which contain information on major disasters, for example, world almanacs, available. There are several published each year and many of them are published in paperback.

Place the following list on the chalkboard:

Cyclones	Volcanic Eruptions
Hurricanes	Floods
Typhoons	Air disasters
Earthquakes	Sea disasters
Avalanches	Rail disasters
Tornados	Fire and Explosion

B. Introduction to the Class: There have been many major disasters in history. I have listed the types on the board. Notice that the weather has caused many of them. Are we subject to any of these in our area? Which ones? What are some of the safety precautions we are taking to help protect us if another disaster should happen? (Continue the discussion according to area, for example, tornado drills at school or dikes for flood control.)

Knowing something about major disasters can help you to understand how important it is to be constantly alert to weather conditions and safety precautions. Today, I would like you to begin a project which will help you gain some insight into the horror of disasters. Use the resource material and research one major disaster in each of the categories listed on the board. Tell what happened, where it happened, how many people were involved, property damage, and if there was something that could have been done to prevent such a disaster.

8. FIRE IN THE FOREST (Grades K-6)

A. Preparation and Materials: Be prepared to discuss forest fires according to grade level.

Example:

Younger children respond well to safety tips from Smokey Bear.

B. Introduction to the Class: Fires are always a danger and forest fires are disasters which destroy thousands of acres of land each year. These fires destroy our natural resources and endanger the lives of animals and people.

Some fires are started by lightning or some other force of nature. There isn't too much we can do about this except to keep a watchful eye out for fires and try to stop them before they get too big.

Some fires are caused by careless campers and others who forget to put out campfires, cigarettes and matches. These are the kinds of forest fires we can help to prevent. We can remember to be very careful with fire.

We can also remember that there are three basic ways to put out a fire. They are:

1. Take away its fuel.
2. Take away its air. (Smother it.)
3. Cool it with water or fire-extinguisher chemicals.

(Continue the discussion according to grade level.)

I know a game called "Fire in the Forest". Let's play it to help us remember what we have learned about forest fire safety.

C. Directions:

1. I will choose one child to be "It". "It" will stand in the center of the circle.

2. The other children will choose a partner. Form a double circle around "It". Players in the outer circle stand directly behind their partner.

3. When "It" calls, "Fire in the Forest, Run, Run, Run!" The players on the outside circle begin to run around the circle.

4. "It" and the players on the inside circle clap their hands.

5. When "It" stops clapping, he and the inside players hold their hands over their heads. This is the signal for the outside players to try to get in front of an inside player.

6. "It" also, tries to find a partner. The player left without a partner becomes the new "It" for the next game.

9. KEYS TO PREPAREDNESS
(Grades 4-8)

A. Preparation and Materials: Have resource material on disasters, their causes, effects, and occurrences and the means for coping with them available.

Examples:

Encyclopedias, geography texts, government publications such as: "Disaster Preparedness, Report to Congress," 1972, Public Documents Distribution Center, 5801 Tabor Ave., Philadelphia, Pennsylvania, 19120.

You will also need crayons and use of a bulletin board. Make a large outline map of the world. **Suggestion:** Use an opaque projector and blow up a map on butcher paper. Outline with black felt pen.

B. Introduction to the Class: Many of the major disasters are caused by the weather. Can you name some of these?

Examples:

Tornados, floods, hurricanes, snowstorms, cyclones, typhoons, avalanches.

These disasters do not occur every place in the world. For example, if you live in North Dakota, you would not expect a hurricane. However, if you lived in Florida, you would know that you must prepare for these storms.

Let's make a color key of these weather caused disasters. Yellow will be the key color for hurricanes. Red will be the color for tornados, etc.

Use the resource material and find out where these weather-caused disasters occur most often in the world. Color that section of the map according to the color key we have made. Remember that some areas of the world are subject to more than one type of storm. Michigan has three types of storms which can cause major disasters. They are tornados, floods and snowstorms. This area of the country must be colored three colors. (Construction paper circles in appropriate colors could be cut and pasted on the map.)

Knowing what to expect where you live is important to your safety. Knowing how to prepare for expected disasters is also very important. I am going to divide the class into groups. Each group will research one type of disaster. Color key your report to match the color of the disaster on the map.

Sample Research Questions:

1. What safety precautions can be taken by individuals?

2. What safety precautions are taken by government?

C. Correlation: Correlate this activity with a geography unit or incorporate it with a study on government.

** **10. CIVIL DEFENSE VOCABULARY (Grades 4-8)**

A. Preparation and Materials: Prepare a duplicated sheet similar to the example. Students will need dictionaries and pencils.

Example:

Defense
_____

_____

**This activity is available in Prevent Volume II of the Spice™ Duplicating Masters.

Survival _____

Edible _____

Conelrad _____

Continue in this way with words, such as mobilization, radiation, emergency, disaster, nuclear, corrosive, evacuation, shielding, fallout, hazard, international, tornado, flash flood, flood, hurricane, civil, sanitary.

B. Introduction to the Class: The words on this paper are all words which are related to civil defense. You should be able to understand them. First, look over the list and write the meaning of each word you already know. Then use your dictionary to find the meaning of each word you do not know.

**11. FAMILY CHECK LIST (Grades 4-8)

A. Preparation and Materials: Prepare a duplicated sheet similar to the example.

Example:

FAMILY CHECK LIST

                                          YES   NO
1. Do all the members in your family know what to do in case of fire, flood, hurricane tornado and nuclear attack?   ____ ____
2. Are your house and yard clear of rubbish?   ____ ____
3. Have your electrical and heating systems been checked for safety?   ____ ____

**This activity is available in Prevent Volume II of the Spice™ Duplicating Masters.

4. Are all fuels and flammable fluids stored in safe containers?   ____ ____

5. Do you have a hand fire extinguisher and/or garden hose located for fire fighting?   ____ ____

6. Do all members of your family know general first aid rules?   ____ ____

7. Has at least one adult in your family had first aid training?   ____ ____

8. Do you have a supply of necessary first aid supplies in your home?   ____ ____

9. Do you have an emergency shelter or space equipped with ample food, water and equipment?   ____ ____

10. Do the members of your family know the warning signals and what to do if they sound?   ____ ____

11. Do you know the protective measures to be used in case of fallout?   ____ ____

12. Is your car kept in good running condition with at least a half a tank of gas in it?   ____ ____

B. Introduction to the Class: We have no control over the weather and very little over international politics. Thus, a disaster could occur anytime. If we know we can't prevent disasters, then it is also important for us to know we can be prepared for it. Being prepared can save lives.

Take this check list home and ask the members of your family to help you answer each question. If your family is prepared, then all of your answers will be "Yes". If you find questions which must be answered "No", perhaps you can encourage your parents to improve the situation.

**12. STORM WARNINGS (Grades 4-8)

A. Preparation and Materials: Have resource material on weather forecasting available. Students will also need notebooks or materials to make notebooks.

B. Introduction to the Class: Learning about the weather can help you be more alert to dangerous storms. For example, what causes a tornado or a hurricane? How would the sky look before one of these storms? If you knew the answers to these questions, you would be better prepared, wouldn't you?

Today, I would like you to start a weather notebook. You may title it "STORM WARNINGS". Use the notebook to start doing some research on severe storms. Watch the newspaper for articles on storms and on weather forecasting. Clip these articles and include them in your notebook.

Let's list some questions for research on the board. Think of things that would be helpful to know about storms. For example, have you ever wondered what causes lightning or snow?

You might also ask and answer questions about the weather that you think are interesting. Have you ever wondered why hurricanes are given girl's names?

**This activity is available in Prevent Volume II of the Spice™ Duplicating Masters.

Examples of Additional Research Questions:

How was the U.S. weather bureau started?
Which President made it a reality?
Can man avert hurricanes and tornados?
What information is required to forecast the weather?
Why is the weatherman often wrong?

SECTION IX: Looking To The Future

All children are interested in their future.
They want to know about things that will
concern them and this section is designed to
help them look forward to a safe future. Some
activities will present safety ideas on high
interest and familiar topics, such as driving a
car, hunting and sky diving. Other activities
are planned to introduce less familiar safety
precautions like insurance, community service
organizations and voting.

**1. INTERNATIONAL COLOR MATCH (Grades 4-8)

A. Preparation and Materials: Prepare a duplicated sheet similar to the example. The students will need pencils.

Example:

INTERNATIONAL COLOR MATCH GAME		
RED		1. General warning.
GREEN		2. Construction and maintenance warning.
YELLOW		3. Services for motorists like camping areas.
ORANGE		4. Prohibitions that must be obeyed like STOP and DO-NOT-ENTER.
BLUE		5. Regulatory signs like speed limits.
BROWN		6. Shows permitted movement.
WHITE		7. Indicates recreational facilities and scenic areas.

(Answers: 4-6-1-2-3-7-5)

B. Introduction to the Class: As a part of an international system to make driving easier and safer, new signs are gradually going up around the world. In 1966 the United States adopted a standard for all our roads and streets. (Federal Highway Safety Act — 1966.)

Many of these new signs use pictures and symbols instead of words. Do any of you know why this would be easier and safer? Yes, Matt. We could travel to another country and know what traffic control signs mean even if we couldn't speak or read the language. It would be the same for visitors to this country.

Lettering on older road signs cannot be easily changed to symbols, but now many road signs have new colors and shapes which will mean the same all over the world. For example, a red sign will indicate a prohibition that must be obeyed.

**This activity is available in Prevent Volume II of the Spice™ Duplicating Masters.

You might not recognize the word "Stop", but if you saw a red, octagon-shaped sign, you could be pretty sure that is what is meant.

Today, let's see if you can figure out what color matches which traffic control. Try the International Color Match Game. When you are finished, we will go over it together. (More time could be given and students could ask the help of their parents or other grown ups.)

**2. INTERNATIONAL SHAPE MATCH (Grades 4-8)

A. Preparation and Materials: The International Shape Match is a follow-up activity to the International Color Match. Prepare a duplicated sheet as follows. The students will need pencils.

Example:

OCTAGON	⬡	
DIAMOND	◇	
PENTAGON	⬠	
RECTANGLE	▭	
PENNANT	▷	
INVERTED TRIANGLE	▽	

1. Means warning.
   Example: SLIPPERY WHEN WET
2. Signals regulations.
   Example: DO NOT ENTER
3. NO PASSING.

This activity is available in Prevent Volume II of the **Spice™ Duplicating Masters.

4. School nearby.
   Example: SCHOOL CROSSING
5. Always means STOP.
6. Means YIELD.

(Answers: 5-1-4-2-3-6)

B. Introduction to the Class: Yesterday, we discussed the importance of color in relation to the international traffic control system. Do you remember that I mentioned also that shapes would play an important role. Today, you are going to try your hand at another match game using shapes and their meanings. Find the definition for the octagon. Put the number into the box opposite the octagon.

You have seen many of these signs. How observant are you? What is the shape of the SCHOOL CROSSING sign?

3. IF I'D BEEN DRIVING (Grades 4-8)

A. Preparation and Materials: Sometimes, one of the best methods for helping students become more aware of safety is to go at it with a high interest adult approach. All students have a high interest in driving and the independence it promises. This activity capitalizes on this and the result is a greater awareness of automobile safety in general.

The students will need to make scrapbooks or buy notebooks. They will also need pencils, scissors and daily newspapers.

B. Introduction to the Class: Someday, most of you will be driving your own car. How many are planning to take driver's training? Driving will give you greater independence, but it also places greater responsibilities on you. Being prepared for these greater responsibilities is one of the best ways to become safer drivers.

Today, you are going to start an "If I'd Been Driving" scrapbook. You will have several days (or a certain number of weeks) to complete this project. Start going through the newspaper. Clip all of the articles you can find on traffic accidents. I'm sure you will have no trouble finding plenty. Paste the clipping in your scrapbook and then write a short paragraph on what you think might have happened. You might consider the following questions:

1. Could the accident have been avoided? How?

2. Are there factors which might have prevented bodily injury?

4. VOTE FOR SAFETY (Grades 6-8)

A. Preparation and Materials: This activity can best be done during the weeks before an election. The students will need campaign literature, pencils and paper.

B. Introduction to the Class: As you know, the _____ elections are coming up. You have probably read or heard something about it. It will be a few years before you can vote in this type of election, but now is not to early to start thinking about how your vote can someday guard your safety.

Many citizens do not know how to vote. They pick a name on the ballot which sounds nice or they may decide to vote for someone just because they like their looks. Do you think this is intelligent voting? Why not?

When you vote for a candidate, you want to know that the person will do the best for you and your community. Intelligent voting takes time, but it is time well spent.

On election day we are going to hold mock elections in our room. Between now and then I would like you to practice some intelligent voting habits.

What do you think would be an intelligent voting habit to develop? Let's make a list on the board.

Sample List:

1. Investigate the candidates qualifications.

2. Study the records. Has the candidate done anything in the past to promote a safer community?

3. Listen to campaign speeches and consider what is being said. Are there any safety claims being made?

4. Determine which candidate you feel is more honest and more intelligent.

5. Decide which candidate you feel will do the most for you and your community.

As you begin investigating the issues and candidates in the election, put your thoughts on paper. Why have you selected a certain person?

On election day you may cast your vote. We will compare our classroom results with the actual results.

C. Variation: The class could become more involved by selecting candidates and making posters and speeches which would support their choices.

5. INTERVIEW A CANDIDATE
(Grades 6-8)

A. Preparation and Materials: Students will need pencils and paper. If possible, set up an interview with a local candidate. This might be done by phone if a personal interview can't be arranged.

B. Introduction to the Class: Today, we are going to think about some questions we could ask _____ .
He/She is running for the office of _____ .
Let's concentrate on safety. For example, what would this candidate say he/she would do about crime in the streets? Should he/she have something in mind considering the office he/she is running for?
Can you think of some other safety concerns?

Examples:
1. Highway safety
2. Gun laws
3. Garbage collection
4. Flood control
5. Safety in the schools
6. Traffic control
7. Airport safety
8. Park safety
9. Laws governing the safe use of recreational vehicles, such as boats, snowmobiles and campers.

6. PAPER CRYSTAL BALLS (Grades 4-8)

A. Preparation and Materials: Each student will need a large circle cut from 12x18 inch white construction paper. They will also need access to a felt pen for labeling, paste, scissors and crayons.

The following list of ideas may be placed on the chalkboard:

sky diving	fishing
skin diving	boating
surfing	water skiing
racing	snow skiing
cars	ballooning
horses	flying a plane
motorcycles	trailbike riding
snowmobiles	dune buggies

B. Introduction to the Class: If you had a gypsy crystal ball and could look into your future, what do you think you would see yourself doing in your leisure time? I've listed several ideas on the board. Can you think of others?

I can't give you a real crystal ball, but I am giving you a paper crystal ball. You project into your future and decide which one of the leisure time activities interests you most. Draw a picture of you doing it, or you may cut a picture of someone else doing it and pretend it is you. Paste it onto the paper ball. Then, find out as much as you can about the safety involved in doing what you have selected. Write a report on this and staple it to the bottom of your picture.

C. Bulletin Board Idea:

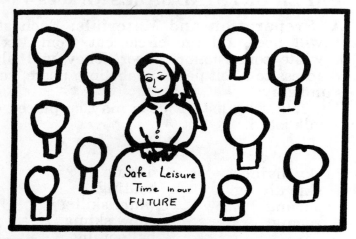

7. SAFETY CAREERS (Grades 6-8)

A. Preparation and Materials: Resource materials available at the school library or public library. Many librarians will assemble materials upon request and have them ready for students. Students might also be encouraged to contact the local chapter of the Red Cross, school counselors, police and fire departments or other safety organizations active in the community.

B. Introduction to the Class: Most of you have given some thought to what you want to do when you grow up. Some of you will change your mind several times between now and the time when you will make a firm decision and there is certainly nothing wrong in changing your mind. In fact, it is good for you to explore careers so that eventually you can make an intelligent decision on one which will bring you the most satisfaction out of life.

Today, you are going to begin a study of the

wide variety of careers in the area of safety. By exploring, you will learn just what careers are available and someday you may decide that one of them appeals to you.

Use the library and research at least ten possible safety careers. Almost any area that interests you could possibly involve a safety career.

You may write your report similar to the example on the board. You may not be able to find exact figures for a projected salary or positions available, but you should get some idea by talking with your parents, school counselors or by calling one of the safety organizations or businesses in the community.

Example of Report Form:

I. (Name of the career.)

    A. (Brief job description.)

    B. (Education Required.)

    C. (Expected salary at the present time.)

    D. (Projected numbers of positions available.)

8. STRAIGHT SHOOTERS (Grades K-6)

A. Preparation and Materials: Make a string or chalk circle on the floor. The "hunters" will need five marbles of one color. Place a handful of other marbles in the center of the circle.

B. Introduction to the Class: One sport many boys and girls look forward to doing when they grow up is hunting. Some of you may go hunting now with your parents. (Continue discussion letting children describe hunting trips.)

One of the first safety rules for hunting is to be sure of your target. Many accidents are caused by hunters who get excited and shoot at anything that moves.

Today, we are going to play a fun game with marbles. This game will help you remember that one of the most important rules for hunting safety is to be sure of your target.

C. Directions:

1. This is the woods. It is our target. (Point to the ring on the floor with the marbles inside it.) The marbles are the game we are hunting, deer, ducks, elk, fox, rabbits, pheasant, moose, bear, squirrel, etc.

2. Each hunter will get five marbles. These are your bullets. If you drop them on the floor before it is your turn, you are out of the game because you are a careless hunter and careless hunters are not safe hunters. When it is your turn, aim carefully. Be sure of your target.

3. The hunter who knocks the most game clear out of the woods (circle) is the winner.

9. COURT IMPRESSIONS (Grades 7-8)

A. Preparation and Materials: Arrange for the class to visit a traffic court in which a case is being tried. Afterwards, the students will need paper and pencils to write their impressions.

B. Introduction to the Class: I have arranged for you to visit a traffic court. A case will be in progress. I would like you to see court proceedings as to how justice is administered to traffic law violators.

When we return, I will ask you to write your impressions. Here are a few questions you might keep in mind.

Sample Questions:

1. Can you see how the court system contributes to safety in our society?
2. Do you think you saw a fair trial?
3. What were your impressions regarding the judge, the defendant, witnesses, arresting officer, etc.?
4. Does the traffic violation seem valid? Why?
5. How did you feel about the fine or lack of one?

C. Correlation: This activity could be used along with a study of government and the court system. Safety could be discussed along with a field trip to view trials other than traffic violations.

10. MOBILE HOME SAFETY (Grades 7-8)

A. Preparation and Materials: Write or call your county or state civil defense office and request the booklet on how to protect mobile homes from high winds. Additional information may be obtained from mobile home manufacturers and sales representatives. The students will need safety notebooks or paper and pencils.

B. Introduction to the Class: More and more adults are buying mobile homes these days. Can you think why this might be true? (Continue discussion as time and interest permits.)

Some of you may decide someday that mobile home living is for you. If you do buy a mobile home, you should be aware of safety precautions which apply especially to mobile home owners. High winds do a great deal of damage to mobile homes each year. Our local civil defense office provides this booklet which tells you how to protect your home.

In your spare time, take a look at the material on mobile home safety and then write a paragraph or two about it in your safety notebook or as an assignment to be handed in. Be sure to include the name of the booklet. Writing it down can help you remember where you might get a copy if you should ever need it in the future.

C. Correlation: This activity could be correlated with an English lesson on paragraphing or material condensation.

**11. AYE AYE, CAPTAIN (Grades 4-8)

A. Preparation and Materials: Make a duplicated sheet similar to the example. Students will need pencils.

This activity is available in Prevent Volume II of the **Spice™ Duplicating Masters.

Example:

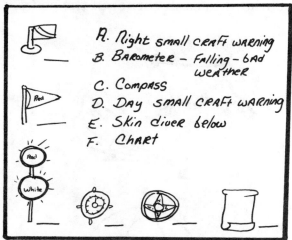

A. Right small craft warning
B. Barometer - Falling - bad weather
C. Compass
D. Day small craft warning
E. Skin diver below
F. Chart

(Answers: E-D-A-B-C-F)

B. Introduction to the Class: Some of you may decide to be the captain of your own boat someday. You will, of course, want to take a boating safety course first. Some states require that you do.

Today, just for fun, see how many of the boating safety symbols you can match. If you get all six right, you can start saving your money for a boat. You have a good start on being a very safe captain. If you miss more than two, you had better ride with another captain until you can take a course in boating safety.

12. SAFETY CHUTES (Grades 4-8)

A. Preparation and Materials: Make or have students make a simple parachute. You will need a square silk scarf, four cords about three feet long and an empty spool.

Directions:

1. Tie cord to each corner of the scarf.

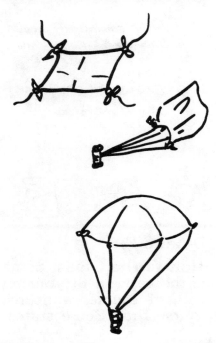

2. Attach the spool to the ends of the four cords.

3. Fold the scarf and throw it as high as you can.

B. Introduction to the Class: If it were possible to look into the future, some of you might see yourself as forest rangers, sky divers or jet race car drivers. These three activities have one very important safety device in common. Can you think what that safety device might be? (Continue discussion, giving clues until parachute is mentioned.)

Leonardo da Vinci made this important safety discovery back in 1495, but it wasn't until 1783 that the first successful jump was made by Louis Sebastian Leonarmand, a Frenchman.

Parachutes were adopted as standard airplane safety equipment by both Britain and the United States during World War II. Many lives were saved as a result.

Since the war, the parachute has found various other uses. We mentioned three earlier. Maybe you can think of others.

Watch this simple parachute demonstration and see if you can tell how a parachute works.

13. INSURANCE SAFETY (Grades 6-8)

A. Preparation and Materials: Invite an insurance man to visit your classroom to discuss insurance and safety.

B. Introduction to the Class: Today, we are going to discuss insurance and safety. I have invited Mr. _____ of the _____ Insurance Company to visit and answer some of our questions.

Sample Questions:

1. Explain the different types of insurance, such as car, hospital, disability, life, fire, homeowners, etc.

2. Does a person always have to die before life insurance pays off?

3. Explain why insurance companies are concerned with safety.

4. What are some of the specific safety programs the insurance company engages in?

5. What do insurance companies do with all of the money they collect?

14. PROBLEM SOLVERS (Grades 4-8)

A. Preparation and Materials: Watch the newspaper and clip two or three examples of new inventions or laws designed to improve automobile safety.

B. Introduction to the Class: A man named Henry Wells was involved in the first automobile accident ever recorded. The accident happened in New York City in 1896. Henry was driving a Duryea Motor Wagon. He collided with a bicycle rider named Evelyn Thomas. Evelyn had to go to the hospital to be treated for a fractured leg. Henry went to jail until a full report could be made.

Since that time, automobile accidents have become one of the number one killers in the country. Why do you suppose this has happened? (More cars, faster, bigger, better roads, etc.)

Can you think of anything that is being done to prevent or reduce the problem? Yes, seatbelts were invented for the sake of safety. The air bag may provide another answer. (Continue discussion and read the examples you have clipped.)

C. Directions: Start watching the newspaper. Ask your parents to help. Look for news regarding new safety devices on automobiles, roads, or laws designed to cut down on auto accidents. When you find something, clip it and bring it to school. We will discuss it and decide if we feel it will help to solve the problem.

D. Variation: Use the clippings as a basis for a bulletin board or classroom booklet on automobile safety.

Students could be asked to try and think up their own invention or law and write a paper on why they think it will help.

15. KNOW YOURSELF (Grades 7-8)

A. Preparation and Materials: Pencils and paper will be needed.

B. Introduction to the Class: Have you ever heard anyone say that someone else is "accident prone?" Do you believe that there are people like this? (Allow students to express their feelings and draw conclusions about this question.)

Some safety experts claim that certain essential elements must be present before an accident can occur. They call this accident sequence. These elements include the person injured, the emotional climate, the object involved in the injury and the physical environment. When all of these elements coincide at the right (or wrong) moment, an accident happens. Can you decide which one of these elements you might have some control over to prevent an accident? Right, the emotional climate is one element you can control if you are aware of how you react under certain situations. This is probably the major element which separates the "accident prone" people from the majority of people who do manage to understand themselves and their reactions.

All people have feelings of anger, worry, fear, stress and tension, but all people do not react the same. Once you have gained some awareness of your strengths and weaknesses, you will know when you should take extra precautions.

Today, I would like you to begin keeping a record of your reactions. For the next few days I will give you about ten minutes before class begins to think about yourself and what you did under certain conditions. I think some of you may be surprised at what you learn about yourself.

**16. ACCIDENT ATTITUDES
(Grades 7-8)

A. Preparation and Materials: Prepare a duplicated sheet of true and false questions similar to those given in the example below. The students will need pencils.

Example:

1. _____ Emotional outbursts could cause accidents.
2. _____ People who are especially happy never cause accidents.
3. _____ Showing-off is a mistaken form of trying to prove oneself.
4. _____ One of the best ways to handle emotional upsets is to talk about them.
5. _____ Frustrations should never be talked out with adults.

Write a brief paragraph using an example to explain each answer.

(T)   (F)   (T)   (T)   (F)

B. Introduction to the Class: We have been doing a lot of talking about accidents and how they can be prevented. Today, I am giving you a paper to do which involves a subject which some people seldom think about in regard to accidents . . . your emotions.

Read the questions carefully and answer

**This activity is available in Prevent Volume II of the Spice™ Duplicating Masters.

them with a T for true and a F for false. Then, explain your answer at the bottom of the paper. You may use examples. When you have finished, we will check the papers together and discuss your answers in class.

17. ASSIGNMENT COURAGE
(Grades 4-8)

A. Preparation and Materials: The purpose of this activity is to give students a basis for drawing on their inner resources if they should become involved in a serious accident in the future. If the assignment is to be written rather than oral, students will need pencils and paper.

B. Introduction to the Class: Accidents can happen to anyone and sometimes they happen in spite of all the safety precautions you may take. Today, I am going to tell you a true story about a man who was involved in a hunting accident six hours before his 18th birthday. His name is Duane Fischer and his accident left him blind. Mr. Fischer could have given up and said the accident ruined his life, but he didn't. Through courage and determination he learned to be self-supporting. He is now married and has a family. He tells everyone he meets that yesterday cannot be changed. Tomorrow cannot be predicted, so one must do the best with what he has got today.

Duane Fischer has magic today. He studied from taped books and practices constantly. As a result he is believed to be the only blind magician in the world. He is a good magician, too. In fact, he is so professional that some have doubted that he is blind at all. He gives many performances a year. Many of them are in elementary schools where he amazes the students with his many feats of magic. He uses the story of his hunting accident as the basis of safety talks which he weaves into his magic show.

Can any of you think why I told you this story? Yes, I think it is important for you to know that if you should be involved in a serious accident someday which leaves you handicapped that you should not give up hope.

Your safety assignment this week will be to keep your eyes and ears open for other stories of courage. Find out what type of accident happened and what handicap resulted and then describe how that person has had the courage to go on and find new meaning for his or her life.

Perhaps you know someone in your own family or neighborhood. You might find an example in the newspaper or hear of someone on television. You might also ask the librarian to suggest some appropriate biographies.

Examples:

1. Glen Cunningham — burned in a fire — track star.

2. Ben Hogan — car accident — famous golfer.

18. GROWING PAINS (Grades K-8)

A. Preparation and Materials: Think of an example of a "growing pains" story from your life which the children would enjoy. It should illustrate the point of this activity which is the chance of an accident is greater when a person does not know how to do something well. For example: a fall when you didn't know how to ride a bike well. As skill increases the chance of an accident decreases.

B. Introduction to the Class: As you grow up, you will be doing many more things. What are some of the things you can do when you grow up that you can't do now?

You can't do some of these things now because it wouldn't be safe. How do you think grown-ups do so many things safely? Many of your parents work at dangerous jobs. How do they avoid accidents? (Discuss several occupations.)

Everything you do increases your chances of an accident, but most grown-ups guard their safety by following one very important safety rule. No matter what they do, they know they must do it well in order to prevent accidents. Can you see how doing things well can decrease the chances for an accident? (Discuss work, play, vacations, sports, driving, etc.)

So it doesn't really matter how many things you do when you grow up or even what kinds of things you choose to do. The important thing to remember is that whatever you do you should always try to know everything you can about it and try to do it well. This is the only safe and happy way to live.

Today, let's prove this by sharing some of our own accident experiences caused by doing something we didn't know how to do very well. For example: (Give your experience.)

19. SAFETY STYLE SHOW (Grades 4-8)

A. Preparation and Materials: Students will need examples of current fashions. Most of what they need can probably be brought from home. Fashion show music (any appropriate record could be used) and a record player. A microphone would be an asset but not a necessity. After the students have put together a show, arrange to present it to another class or schedule a school assembly and present it to the entire school.

B. Introduction to the Class: Fashions in clothes, hair and shoes can affect safety. Can you give some examples? What about high heel shoes or shoes with platforms? Can wide-leg pants affect safety? How? Sun glasses at night may be fashionable but are they safe? (Continue discussion and list possibilities for fashion show on the board.)

We have quite a list of fashions that might affect safety on the board. We can add more later if we think of something but now I think it would be fun if we started to make plans for a safety style show. We could do it like any other style show with one exception. As you model a certain fashion, we will explain how it may be unsafe and then show it can be safe or suggest some precautions to take.

Let's make a list of some things we will need for our show. We will then divide the class into teams and begin work.

Suggestions: They will need to select a script committee, a music selector, a committee to organize and gather appropriate fashions, models and a narrator. Scenery could also be made simple or complex.

** 20. FUTURE SAFETY VOCABULARY (Grades 4-8)

A. Preparation and Materials: Prepare a duplicated sheet similar to the example or put the word list on the chalkboard. Students will need pencils and dictionaries.

**This activity is available in Prevent Volume II of the Spice™ Duplicating Masters.

Example:

Protection
_____

Adjustment
_____

Responsibility
_____

Intoxicated
_____

Additional words for study are examination, politician, candidate, campaign, zoning, and primaries.

B. Introduction to the Class: The words on this paper are all words related to safety in your future. Some day you will be voting on safety laws that will affect you and your family. What does "campaign" mean?

When you buy insurance can you say what "protection" and "adjustment" mean?

All of these words are words which you should understand. First, look over the list and write the meaning of any words you already know. Then, use your dictionary to find the meaning of each word you do not know.

SECTION X: Review and Reinforcement Activities

The ideas and activities in this section are general. They can be used, as the title suggests, for review or for reinforcement as many areas of safety could be briefly covered in each activity. Some teachers may wish to use these ideas when their time for specific safety lessons is limited and they want to cover as much as possible in a short period of time.

1. SAFETY PEEP SHOW (Grades 4-8)

A. Preparation and Materials: The children will need a shoe box for each group of three or four children. They will also need crayons, construction paper, glue, scissors, wax paper or clear plastic wrap and other items of scenery which they can decide upon and collect.

The teacher may want to make a sample peep show box to stimulate ideas. Directions are as follows:

1. Select a scene idea, such as what to do in case of fire or how to prevent (or cause) a fall.

2. Glue a colored background at one end of the box.

3. Cut a peep hole at the other end.

4. Tape a wax paper or plastic wrap window in the top of the lid and hold the box beneath a light when viewing the safety scene inside.

Example:

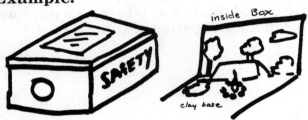

B. Introduction to the Class: The class has been divided up into groups. Each group will decide upon a peep show idea similar to the example I've shown you. If your group has trouble thinking of something, come to me and I will help you get started. You may use any of the supplies I have here and you may want to bring some special things from home. Just be sure it will fit into your shoebox.

Next Wednesday will be peep show day.

2. SAFETY FLAGS (Grades 3-8)

A. Preparation and Materials: The children will need something to use for their flagpole. It could be dowels, flat cardboard, unsharpened pencils or twigs. Other supplies needed are cloth or paper scraps, scissors and glue.

B. Introduction to the Class: We know many safety symbols. (Stop sign, Smokey Bear, Skull and Cross Bones, Railroad Crossing, etc.) Today, you might like to create your own safety symbol. This symbol can be made on your own personal flag.

Later, you will have a chance to show your flag and you may like to discuss the meaning of your symbol.

C. Directions:

1. You may use any shape for your flag. It can be a square, a rectangle, a triangle, a circle or even a free form.

2. When you have decided on your background, cut out the symbol you want to go on your personal flag. Glue in place.

3. Next, glue the flag to the stick by putting glue along one edge of the back side of the flag. Then place the stick on the glued part.

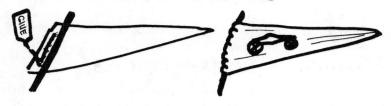

Let it dry. Then, add on more glue and wrap the flag around the stick on a complete turn.

3. PANTOMIME PARTY GAME
(Grades K-8)

A. Preparation and Materials: Select several familiar and easy to act out safety slogans or sayings. Put them on index cards so the teams can take turns drawing them out. (They may be whispered to younger children.)

B. Directions to the Class: Can you guess what I am doing? Yes, I am looking both ways before I cross a street. Today, we are going to divide up in teams and play a pantomime game like this. I have several safety slogans and sayings in this box. When it is your team's turn, one person from your team will draw a card from the box. Read it and then, when I say "Go", that person will have one minute to pantomime the saying on the card. If the team guesses it, they will get one point. If someone from another team guesses and says it out loud, they will have one point subtracted from their score.

When all of the cards are gone, the game is over and I will give a prize to the team with the most points.

Prize Suggestions:

A raisin, marshmallow or small candy.

A few minutes of free time or release from some assigned task.

A star or sticker.

4. ADVERTISING SAFETY (Grades 4-8)

A. Preparation and Materials: Art and writing supplies should be available in the classroom.

B. Introduction to the Class: If you had something you wanted to sell, how would you go about it?

Yes, you would advertise and there are many ways to advertise. Let's make a list on the board.

Example:

Newspapers
Radio
T.V.
Billboards
Posters in store windows
Sandwich men
Word of mouth

People want to advertise things they feel are important. We have decided in this class that safety is important to us and those around us so let's start an advertising campaign for safety. Look at the list on the board. Decide how you would like to advertise a safety idea that you feel is especially important and then go to work on your advertisement. When you have finished, we will use your work to remind everyone in the school (community) about safety.

5. SAFETY POSTER PUZZLES
(Grades K-3)

A. Preparation and Materials: Collect a series of safety posters. (Many organizations and companies provide free safety materials for schools.) Glue the posters onto tagboard. Laminate for longer lasting puzzles. Next, cut the posters using an average of about two or three cuts. This is usually plenty for younger children. Put puzzles in individual boxes or folders.

Example:

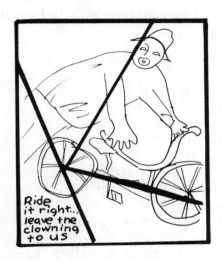

Ride it right... leave the clowning to us

B. Introduction to the Class: I have made some new puzzles for you to work in your spare time. These are very special puzzles. They are safety puzzles and when you have completed one, you will be reminded of some safety rule we have discussed in class.

When you have finished with your puzzle, be sure to put it back in the box (or folder) so we won't get our special puzzle pieces mixed up.

6. SAFETY SCAVENGER HUNT
(Grades K-2)

A. Preparation and Materials: Write each letter of the word S A F E T Y on two index cards so that you have two sets of six cards each.

B. Introduction to the Class: We have been talking about safety and we know that we must think about safety almost all of the time. We should also know how to spell the word "safety" so today we are going to play a match game that will help us remember.

First, you will close your eyes. Then, I will hide one set of cards with the safety letters on them around the room. Next, I will give six of you a card. Your card will have a safety letter on it, too. Now, you must look around the room and match your letter to another one that looks just like it. If you find one that doesn't match, leave it alone and look someplace else. When you have your card matched, go and stand in front of the room. When all six of you are up there, you can arrange the cards to spell the word "safety". I have printed it on the board to help you remember how it goes.

When all of the letters are matched and the word is spelled, you may give your card to someone else and we will play the game again with six different people.

*7. SAFETY SUBTRACTION (Grades 1-4)

A. Preparation and Materials: Trace or draw safety ideas on to a duplicating master. The pictures should be fairly simple to color. Put a subtraction fact on each object to be colored. Include a number key as shown in the illustration. The children will need crayons and perhaps a piece of scrap paper to figure the answers.

*This activity is available in Prevent Volume I of the Spice™ Duplicating Masters.

Example:

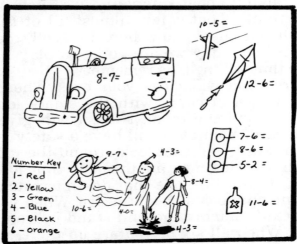

B. Directions to the Class: This activity is a little like painting by numbers, except you will have to figure out the numbers by using your math facts. Notice at the bottom of the page I have put a number key; 1-Red, 2-Yellow, etc. Look at the pictures. All of them show some safety idea we have talked about in class. There is a number sentence on each picture or picture part. Solve the problem and then you will know which color to use. As you color, try to think of the safety rules we discussed.

8. TAPE TALKS AND SAFETY SKITS (Grades K-8)

A. Preparation and Materials: An interesting method for reinforcing and reviewing safety lessons is to allow students to tape talks and safety skits. A tape recorder and tape are all that is needed.

B. Introduction to the Class: We have discussed many safety ideas and I'm sure all of you have learned a great deal. Today, you may get into groups or you may work alone if you would like. Select a safety idea which you think is important and prepare a talk or skit about it. Then, I would like you to tape it. When your tape is finished, we will have a presentation period so the whole class can share your idea.

Here are some talk and skit suggestions you may want to use.

1. Watch Out For Dangerous Toys — Direct attention to the danger of games, such as darts, archery sets, skate boards, toys with small plastic parts, bikes and swinging yoyos. The skit could suggest safe ways of using these toys and games.

2. Swimming Safety — This skit could focus on a scene at the beach or pool where children discuss rules for swimming.

3. A-Hunting We Will Go — Talk about gun safety — what to do if you get lost — what to do if you see someone shot or having a heart attack.

4. Friendly Strangers Aren't Always Friendly — Discuss what to do if a stranger tries to pick you or another youngster up.

9. SAFETY PUPPETS (Grades K-8)

A. Preparation and Materials: Another effective method for making safety lessons interesting is to have students make puppets. Puppets used should be simple so that they can be constructed easily and so that the emphasis of the activity remains on the content of the material presented.

Materials needed are cloth or heavy paper, yarn, needle, fabric scraps or felt pens, glue, newspaper and a simple pattern.

Example:

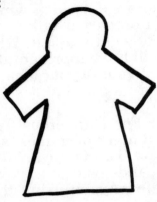

B. Introduction to the Class: Today, we are going to make safety puppets. We are going to make very simple puppets so that we can make them quickly and give more time to our safety skits.

C. Directions:

1. Cut a pattern from newspaper by folding the paper in half and cutting the shape shown in the example.

2. Test the length and width to make sure it will cover your hand. Allow plenty of room so you will be able to move your puppet.

3. Place pattern on the cloth or heavy paper and cut out.

4. Stitch around puppet. Be sure to leave the bottom open so you can put your hand inside.

5. Scraps of cloth or felt may be glued on for eyes, nose and mouth or you may use a felt pen to draw the features.

D. Additional Skit Ideas:

1. Holiday Haunts: Rules for a safe Christmas tree and lights could be explained, combustibles near a fireplace, what to do with wrapping paper after the gifts are opened, holiday parties, keep sidewalks clear for guests, leave front light on, check for burning cigarettes after guests leave.

2. Danger Lives in the Living Room: Point out the possible dangers that might be present in any living room, wires under a rug, baby playing with electric cord, matches within reach of small children, ladders used for hanging pictures.

3. Waiting For The Doctor: One accident could be presented in the skit, for example, a boy with a broken leg, a baby who has swallowed aspirin or other poison, someone caught in electrical wires.

4. When The Test Isn't A Test: Explain procedures to be followed if you hear the civil defense warning, at home, at school, while shopping.

10. AROUND THE CLOCK (Grades K-8)

A. Preparation and Materials: Decide on an appropriate color scheme. One idea would be to cover, or have students cover, a bulletin board with black paper. Make a red border. Cut two sets of letters, one red and one yellow. Use the red set for shading the yellow set. The hands of the clock could be done the same way.

Twelve paper plates, drawing paper, crayons, scissors, glue and magazines for cutting safety pictures will be needed.

Example:

B. Introduction to the Class: Each of the twelve paper plates stand for a number on the clock. Today, I would like you to think of some of the things you do or things others should do to be safe around the clock.

You may draw a picture or find a picture in a magazine. Make sure your picture is small enough to be cut and pasted on a paper plate. Some paper plates may have more than one picture on them. For example, if two or three of you find a picture (or make one) on fire safety, we will fit them on the same paper plate.

Mike, can you think of an idea for one of the plates?

Yes, a picture of stairs without toys on them would be good. It tells us we should keep stairs and walkways clear to prevent falls.

Right, Sally, another good idea would be to have a picture of someone wearing a seat belt in a car. This reminds us that many auto accident injuries could be prevented if people would wear seat belts.

(Continue the discussion until you are sure students have enough ideas to begin the project.)

11. SPOTLIGHT ON SAFETY (Grades K-8)

A. Preparation and Materials: Select a color scheme and arrange to have enough paper to do the bulletin board chosen. The board may be teacher made or student prepared in the older grades.

Example:

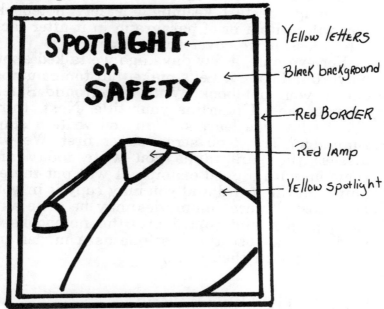

B. Introduction to the Class: We are going to use this bulletin board to display some of our work on safety. Sometimes, we will be displaying safety ideas on specific topics which I have assigned. Other times, you may bring in a clipping from a newspaper or magazine which is related to safety. If you bring something, you will get a chance to tell the class what it is and why you selected it. Then, you may display it in the safety spotlight.

12. SAFETY SUMMARIES (Grades 4-8)

A. Preparation and Materials: Students will need notebooks and pencils. Notebooks could be homemade if you do not wish students to buy them. Start the notebooks early in the school year.

B. Introduction to the Class: Today, you are going to start keeping a safety notebook. You will write a brief paragraph in it after each safety lesson we cover this year.

For example, a few days ago we talked about playground safety. Let's make that topic number one in your notebook. Write Playground Safety on page one. Underline your title. Next, think about what you learned. Can you write a short summary? Try it on scrap paper first. We will discuss the paragraphs you write today and come up with a good example. I will put the example on the board and you may copy it in your notebook. (Future summaries may be done as a class project and copied into the notebooks or students may use the first one as a model and after that write their own.)

13. T.V. TIPS (Grades K-8)

A. Preparation and Materials: Integrate the home T.V. set with safety activities at school. Keep an eye out for up-coming television programs which are safety oriented or those which sound as if safety will be included. Sometimes, specials on specific topics, such as winter sports, water sports, disasters, etc., will include many safety ideas which could be followed up with a discussion the next day at school.

B. Introduction to the Class: Thursday

night Channel _____ will be showing a program called _____ at 7 p.m. Try to watch it and keep your eyes and ears open for safety tips on (the activity). Tomorrow, we will discuss the program in class.

**14. JUST FOR YOU (Grades 4-8)

A. Preparation and Materials: Prepare a duplicated sheet as shown in the example.

Example:

```
7  6  8  3  6  2  3  7  4  6  8  2
S  U  B  U  B  U  P  T  U  E  U  T

8  2  5  6  7  3  4  8  5  8  3  6
C  A  U  S  O  L  S  K  R  L  A  M

8  7  8  6  3  4  8  5  7  6  4  2
E  P  U  A  Y  E  P  W  L  R  C  K

7  4  3  2  3  7  5  4  3  4  2  7
O  A  S  E  A  O  I  U  F  T  E  K

2  4  7  2  4  2  5  6  7  5  4  2
C  I  G  A  O  R  S  T  O  E  N  E
```

DIRECTIONS:
1. Count the letters in your first name.
2. If 6 or more, subtract 4.
3. If less than 6, add 3.
4. Your answer is your safety number.
5. Letters under your number spell a safety message just for you.

B. Introduction to the Class: Today, I am giving you a safety paper to work in your spare time. Read the directions to find your personal safety number. Use the letters under your number to discover a special safety message just for you.

**This activity is available in Prevent Volume II of the Spice™ Duplicating Masters.

C. Variation: Suggest that students might like to experiment with creating their own safety message puzzle using this technique. Caution them to keep messages short. They must also be sure the total number of letters will equal an even number. The example has 60 letters which fit into a 5x12 inch grid.

15. SAFETY DETECTIVES (Grades 3-8)

A. Preparation and Materials: Make a collection of safety points of interest. Keep a card file on them for future reference.

Examples:

1. Museum of old fire fighting equipment, Cincinnati, Ohio, an interesting collection and display of old fire fighting equipment.

2. Unusual Civil Defense shelter, Chattanooga, Tennessee. This shelter is inside Lookout Mountain in the Ruby Falls cave. It is 1,120 feet underground. You must descend in an elevator through 260 feet of solid rock.

3. Safetyville, U.S.A. — Flint, Michigan. A park which includes a miniature safety village. Children may obtain a safety license after learning to drive in miniature cars and taking a written test.

B. Introduction to the Class: There are many safety points of interest around the United States. Be on the lookout for them as you travel on your vacations. Here are some examples from my collection. (Share some interesting places from your file or use the examples above.)

Do any of you have a safety point of interest to share?

Do you think we might have some safety points of interest right here in our own (city) (neighborhood) (state)?

Today, I am going to make all of you safety detectives. The case you are going to solve involves finding as many safety points of interest as you can. When you find one, write name, location and a note or two about it on a file card. The student who finds the most points of interest will be the super safety detective in our class.

C. Correlation: This activity could be used as the basis of an English theme or as an exercise in writing a tour guide correlated with a social studies project.

16. TOTAL SCHOOL PROJECTS
(Grades K-8)

A. Safety Fair

This activity would make a good culminating project for the end of the school year. The gym or all purpose room should be reserved. A principal-teacher committee would be needed to coordinate the fair. Each class in the building could be assigned a safety booth. They could select a certain area of safety and display student work, such as pictures, rule charts, projects and reports. Appropriate demonstrations could be planned for certain time periods. Some classes might give safety skits or present debates or programs.

B. Safety Week

This could be a special week set aside during the school year which is devoted to safety concentration. Appropriate publicity could be arranged. Bulletin boards could be centered on safety. Special assemblies could be held. Guest speakers could be invited.

C. Safety Show Case

A monthly schedule could be set up which would assign each class or grade the hall showcase. Some area of safety could be displayed.

Examples: September — Bike safety, October — Halloween safety, November — Safety in school, December — Christmas tree safety, January — Winter sport safety, February — Fire prevention, March — Kite safety or electric safety, April — Poison prevention, May — Playground safety, June — Vacation safety.

INDEX

DUPLICATOR BOOKS

Use our ideas in duplicator form to cut teacher preparation time and fulfill the needs for supplementary activities in the following areas of study:

LANGUAGE ARTS

- ☐ **ED501-5 SPICE VOL. I** — K-2
- ☐ **ED502-3 SPICE VOL. II** — 2-4
- ☐ **ED505-8 ANCHOR VOL. I** — 4-6
- ☐ **ED506-6 ANCHOR VOL. II** — 6-8
- ☐ **ED564-3 PHONICS VOL. I** — K-2
- ☐ **ED565-1 PHONICS VOL. II** — 2-4
- ☐ **ED567-8 GRAMMAR VOL. I** — 4-6
- ☐ **ED568-6 GRAMMAR VOL. II** — 6-8
- ☐ **ED509-0 RESCUE VOL. I** — K-4
  (Remedial Reading)
- ☐ **ED516-3 FLAIR VOL. I** — 3-8
  (Creative Writing)
- ☐ **ED527-9 DICTIONARY VOL. I** — K-2
  (Single Letters)
- ☐ **ED528-7 DICTIONARY VOL. II** — K-2
  (Blends)
- ☐ **ED529-5 DICTIONARY VOL. III** — 3-6
- ☐ **ED530-9 DICTIONARY VOL. IV** — 7-9
- ☐ **ED537-6 LIBRARY VOL. I** — 3-6
- ☐ **ED538-4 LIBRARY VOL. II** — 7-9

MUSIC

- ☐ **ED561-9 NOTE VOL. I** — K-2
- ☐ **ED562-7 NOTE VOL. II** — 3-6

ONLY $6⁹⁵ Each

EARLY LEARNING

- ☐ **ED512-0 LAUNCH VOL. I**
  (Basic Readiness)
- ☐ **ED513-9 LAUNCH VOL. II**
  (Additional Skills)

MATHEMATICS

- ☐ **ED533-3 PLUS VOL. I** — K-2
- ☐ **ED534-1 PLUS VOL. II** — 2-4
- ☐ **ED523-6 CHALLENGE VOL. I** — 4-6
- ☐ **ED524-4 CHALLENGE VOL. II** — 6-8

SCIENCE

- ☐ **ED546-5 PROBE VOL. I** — K-2
- ☐ **ED547-3 PROBE VOL. II** — 2-4
- ☐ **ED550-3 INQUIRE VOL. I** — 4-8

SOCIAL STUDIES

- ☐ **ED553-8 SPARK VOL. I** — K-2
- ☐ **ED554-6 SPARK VOL. II** — 2-4

* *

DRAMA-PAK™

- Complete play book for each main character and director
- Simple stage settings
- Designed for all ages
- Complete stage directions
- Approximately 15 minutes each

$9⁹⁵

☐ **ED304-7 SCHOOL FOR ANGELS**
A fantasy
Six main characters

☐ **ED300-4 THE WRONGFUL CLAIM**
An old-fashioned melodrama
Eight characters

☐ **ED301-2 THE GRUMBLE GROUP**
A comedy
Five characters

☐ **ED305-5 THE READING OF THE WILL**
A farce
Seven characters

☐ **ED303-9 ME, BETH CONNORS**
A teenage drama
Seven characters

☐ **ED302-0 MR. TEDLEY'S TREEHOUSE**
A drama for the young
Seven characters

For more information contact:

Educational Service, Inc.
Box 219, Stevensville, MI 49127

Toll-Free 1-800-253-0763
Michigan (616) 429-1451

61485